FABULOUS PRAISE
FOR FABULUPUS!

"Lupus is the "disease with a thousand faces". As a physician who treats lupus, this expression resonates with me. Yet, I often observed that it is of little impact to my patients. They are one and for them, lupus has only one face – theirs. When the mirror reflects a teen or young adult, one thousand questions assails them at the time of diagnosis and for years thereafter. This book "Fabulupus: How to be Young, Successful and Fabulous with Lupus", by Nimigon-Young and Kundapur, answers several of these interrogations with the sensibility and relevance that only the experience of living with lupus can give. Thank you for this important work that should be read by persons living with lupus, their families … and their health care team."

Paul R Fortin, MD, MPH, FRCPC
Tenured Professor, Department of Medicine, Laval University
Canadian Research Chair : Systemic Autoimmune Rheumatic Diseases

"A great blueprint for young people struggling with the diagnosis of a chronic illness like lupus. Need help finding your way? Want to be reminded that you're not alone? This book could be your lifeline."

Sara Gorman, author,
Despite Lupus: How to Live Well with a Chronic Illness
www.despitelupus.com

"An outstanding monograph which constructively provides children and their parents a positive, incremental roadmap for coping with a serious disease."

Daniel J Wallace MD
Clinical Professor of Medicine
David Geffen School of Medicine at UCLA

"Jessica and Jodie know from personal experience what it is like to be a young person living with lupus AND still live a meaningful and fun life. Their positive attitudes come through the words on the page in this helpful, easy-to-read book."

Cindy Coney

Speaker and Author of *The Wild Woman's Guide to Living with Illness*

www.cindyconey.com

"I was officially diagnosed with Systemic Lupus Erythematosus at age 14, but had been living with a multitude of its symptoms my entire life. I remember having to make a very difficult choice; I was either going to live with Lupus, or Lupus was going to live with me. I decided the latter was the way to go. I have been running Lupus Awareness campaigns for the last ten years in the form of support groups, walks and more currently, charity motorcycle rides. Books like the one in your hand now have helped me carry on, and have helped me help others. "

Jenn Ephgrave

www.rideforlupus.ca

"Research has shown that young people with lupus face barriers to establishing successful careers. However, they have few places to turn for guidance. Fabulupus provides valuable encouragement and sound advice on finding fulfillment in education, relationships, recreation and the work place."

Dr. Erica Lawson

Pediatric rheumatologist, University of California San Francisco

"Fabulupus is an easy to read guide, both for people with and without lupus. The information in Fabulupus is practical, useful, encouraging, and fun! It reinforces the fact that life does not end with lupus-you can have lupus and still go on to do great things in life and continue to fulfill your dreams."

Florence, a.k.a Miz Flow

Blogger at *The Life of a 20-Something With Lupus*

www.flowonlupus.com

FABULUPUS:

HOW TO BE YOUNG, SUCCESSFUL AND FABULOUS (WITH LUPUS)

JODIE NIMIGON-YOUNG &
JESSICA KUNDAPUR

RANI ROSE PUBLISHING

2014

For information contact
Rani Rose Publishing,
PO BOX 59002 Alta Vista
Ottawa, Canada.
ranirosepublishing@gmail.com

Library and Archives Canada Cataloguing in Publication

Nimigon-Young, Jodie, 1981-, author
Fabulupus : how to be young, successful & fabulous (with lupus) / Jodie
Nimigon-Young & Jessica Kundapur.

Includes index.
Issued in print and electronic formats.
ISBN 978-0-9938494-0-4 (pbk.).--ISBN 978-0-9938494-1-1 (epub)

1. Systemic lupus erythematosus--Popular works. 2. Systemic lupus
erythematosus--Patients. I. Kundapur, Jessica, author II. Title.

RC924.5.L85N55 2014   362.1967'72   C2014-906275-3
                                                   C2014-906276-1

ATTN: QUANTITY DISCOUNTS ARE AVAILABLE TO YOUR ORGANIZATION,
EDUCATIONAL INSTITUTION, OR SUPPORT GROUP
for reselling, educational purposes, subscription incentives, gifts, or
fundraising campaigns.

For more information, please contact the publisher at
Rani Rose Publishing,
PO BOX 59002 Alta Vista
Ottawa, Canada
ranirosepublishing@gmail.com

ABOUT THE AUTHORS

Jodie Nimigon-Young was diagnosed with lupus when she was only
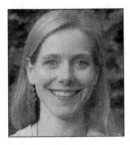 13 years old. Yet, this didn't stop her from accomplishing her goals and dreams. Jodie obtained a Bachelor's degree in Psychology and also obtained a Masters degree in Social Work. Jodie is currently a health care social worker helping patients and families. She lives in Ottawa, Canada with her husband and son.

Jessica Kundapur was diagnosed with lupus when she was 26. Yet,
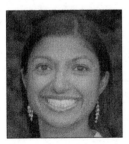 she never gave up on herself or her dreams of having an interesting career and a fantastic life. Jessica completed her Masters degree in biology and began a career in biomedical research. Furthermore, she has lived fabulously with her illness all over the world. She lives in the Netherlands with her husband and daughter.

Jodie's Dedication

This book is dedicated to my parents and sister
for their endless support during my initial diagnosis and my
sometimes stressful adjustment while learning to live a fabulous
life with lupus; to my husband for being with me through the good,
bad and ugly of the writing and publishing process, and
my son for teaching me to appreciate the little things in life.
To all the lupus youth I have encountered over the years
who have inspired me to persevere through the lengthy
and challenging writing process, it is because
of you that I know this book is needed,
and the challenge worthwhile.

Jessica's Dedication

This book is dedicated to my amazing mother for looking
after me every day of my life, my husband who supports
me each day in the present, and my daughter for inspiring
me to create adventure-filled days for the future. And to
all of you with lupus, rest assured, everything will be okay.
In fact, everything will be fabulous.

ACKNOWLEDGEMENTS

Our deepest and sincerest thanks to:

Carolina Pineda for reading the first version of the School & Education chapter and for providing the feedback that guided the rest of the book.

Nathan Rosthoven for volunteering to review several of the chapters and encouraged us to finish the book and get it published.

Kristine Nimigon for reading our early drafts of the chapters, helping us to conceptualize potential formats of the book and inspiring us to continue writing.

Sara Gorman, who provided fantastic practical advice, and gave us the confidence to move forward with publishing this book. Her book: *Despite Lupus: How to Live Well with a Chronic Illness* will enlighten you to a whole new level.
www.despitelupus.com

Andra Weber, for designing a fabulous book cover and the beautiful interior and whose knowledge of publishing and marketing was essential to the creation of this book.
www.andrawebercreative.com

Geoff Whyte for helping to shape the manuscript.
www.whyteink.com.au

Gina Dunn for enthusiastically creating our fun website.
www.igina.net

Various cafés located in Kingston, Montréal, Ottawa, Berkeley and Nijmegen, where these words were typed over many cups of coffee and a few cookies.

Our friends, both local and global, who hung out with us when we were ill, partied with us when were healthy and who always thought that this book was a great idea.

Our families, for looking out for us, taking care of us, and believing in us.

Our respective husbands, for loving us in sickness and in health, encouraging us with this book, traveling with us so that we could meet to discuss and write, reviewing chapters, and for holding our respective babies while we typed.

Finally, to all of you with lupus, your courage inspired us to dream and write.

Jodie Nimigon-Young & Jessica Kundapur

FOREWORD

The moment you're diagnosed with lupus, your mind is flooded with questions that have no concrete answers: What does this diagnosis mean? How will it affect me? What about my plans for the future? Facing the disease as a young person creates an additional layer of unknowns, and that can be downright scary. What you need is a plan to start putting the pieces of your life together, with lupus in tow. You want to know how you're going to keep moving forward, and you want someone to tell you how it can be done. And that's what Jodie and Jessica have done: written an honest, practical, useful book about managing life with lupus geared toward young people. And even better, it's based upon their experiences with the disease.

No matter at what age you're diagnosed, you're searching for answers. I felt that same way the day I was diagnosed with lupus in my mid-twenties. I had been married for six weeks and was at a high point in my television career. I remember asking myself: what if the diagnosis had come just a few months earlier, during my engagement? Or, what if it had happened before we'd even met? What if I was at the beginning of my career, or college-bound, or just entering high school? What obstacles would I have encountered, and how would I have tackled them?

While I never had to search for those answers, I've been asked those questions many times before. As the author of *Despite Lupus*, I share my story with lupus patients throughout the world. I've encountered thousands of people with lupus, and I'm able to provide guidance, based upon my experience, to many of them. But there is a very special group of people to whom I cannot serve as a resource on certain issues – the many young people, both teenagers and young adults, who are diagnosed with this illness.

In this book, young people can learn from the first-hand experience of the authors, who provide not one, but two distinct stories that can motivate, inspire, and provide hope. Theirs may be different. Theirs may be better. Theirs may be worse. But you'll have another set of experiences to draw upon and to remind yourself you're not crazy in the wake of this overwhelming disease called lupus.

The real value of this book is in the honest, reassuring voices of the authors. They candidly tell you what worked for them, and what didn't. They outline steps that led to their successes, and list pitfalls to avoid. Firstly, because the book is a collaboration, they know that not every patient is affected in the same way. Lupus isn't a cookie-cutter disease – so the authors provide options. They offer several ways to deal with and respond to emotional and physical situations that arise, allowing you to tailor your young adult life to lupus.

Secondly, the insights they share come to you via the perspective of a lupus patient, rather than a doctor, family member, or friend, each of whom can only imagine what it's like to walk in your shoes. This first-hand knowledge has a greater impact coming from someone who's actually lived it. There's a familiarity that only exists within the mind of a lupus patient, and it might be a source of support you didn't even know you were missing.

Lastly, you have two examples of success stories, two young ladies who are making their lives work in the face of their disease. Their stories will remind you that you can do this. It is possible. Life with lupus is manageable for any young person like you.

Personally, this book fills a gap in my lupus education. While I might not be able to address young adults on the issues that arise during the formative teenage years, as a single person in the dating world, or as someone trying to balance school with a chronic illness, I now have a valuable navigational tool to share. It's called "Fabulupus: How to be young, successful and fabulous (with lupus)."

With deepest respect,
Sara Gorman
Author, *Despite Lupus: How to Live Well with a Chronic Illness*
www.despitelupus.com
January 14, 2014

CONTENTS

TABLE OF CONTENTS

INTRODUCTION

Why Me?

You are probably reading this book because you have been diagnosed with a crazy-sounding chronic illness called Systemic Lupus Erythematosus. Try saying that 10 times fast! You are confused about what this means, angry about why you were the one diagnosed, and not someone else, and sad about possibly losing some things in your life that are important to you. You are annoyed because your parents are freaking out, and you're scared to talk about your illness with your friends. You are worried about how much your life will change, and whether you can still do all the things you want. We can totally relate, because we have both experienced these same emotions. Jodie was diagnosed with lupus at the age of 13, and Jessica at 26. We have both learned to cope with the challenges of living with a chronic health condition, and thought that other people could relate to and learn from our experiences. Most importantly, we want you to know that you can still have an amazing life with lupus. How do we know? Because we have done it ourselves.

What is Lupus?

As your doctor has hopefully explained, lupus is an autoimmune disorder. This means that your own immune system is attacking different parts of your body. Your immune system usually protects you from harmful viruses and bacteria, but with lupus your immune system is "confused," and fights your own body instead. Your immune system can attack any part of your body, and this is why lupus symptoms can be different in every patient. Lupus can affect any part of your body, but most commonly causes arthritis, rashes, kidney complications, fever, pleurisy, Raynaud's phenomenon, and mouth ulcers. There are also individuals who experience skin, heart, brain, or liver problems. Think about it – lupus can impact any part of your body, and your body is made up of many different, complex parts. Most people experiencing a lupus flare-up feel fatigue, muscle/joint pain, sun-sensitivity, sores in their nose/mouth, chest pain, and hair loss. Other symptoms may develop depending upon what parts of their body are being attacked.

Just so you know, this is basically the extent of the "medical information" that you will find in this book. We understand that you have likely been inundated with medical terms from lots of different people and sources: we don't want to add to that pile of information. The point we are trying to make is that because lupus can attack any part of the body, the illness can be incredibly difficult to manage. Also, you might not know *where* or *when* the lupus will attack, which can cause anxiety and stress. The unpredictability is the worst part about lupus, and flare-ups always seem to happen at the worst possible time. But really, is there a good time for a flare-up to arrive, leaving you sick, exhausted and in pain? No. The unpredictable nature of this disease makes it really hard to plan for things that are important to you, like your schoolwork, or a party, or your friends. But, that doesn't mean that you can't do the things you want, the things you love and the things that you need to do to have a successful life.

A few more facts; lupus is most common in women, with only one man being diagnosed in every 10 patients. Lupus often strikes young adults. Lupus may seem like a very weird chronic illness, but it is actually more common than multiple sclerosis, leukemia and muscular dystrophy combined! This may seem strange, because you have likely heard of these other conditions, but not lupus, until now, but it's true[1]. Even though lots of people are diagnosed with lupus, and many are diagnosed as teenagers or young adults, there's not a lot of information out there to help guide young people to success in managing this condition. This doesn't make any sense to us, because most people with lupus are diagnosed with this crazy, unpredictable illness during the craziest, most unpredictable time of their lives. There is so much going on in your life right now, *plus* you have this new chronic condition, and so you really need to know

---

1 http://www.lupusontario.org/education-and-resources.aspx

how to cope with all the stuff that matters to you.

How Do I Live with Lupus?

When you are newly diagnosed, it can feel like everything is being taken away from you. For instance, you need to sleep a lot more, so you may have to make lifestyle changes like spending less time with your friends, and you may need to stop going to school/work, or even be admitted to hospital, to help your body heal. You will notice that your parents, family and friends will become more protective, and will always be very worried about what you are doing. There are so many changes required, many of them overwhelming. You may need to alter some of your future goals, which can be super frustrating. You may wonder, 'How am I going to live with this illness and still live my life?' It is precisely because of experiencing these same thoughts and emotions that we have teamed up to write this book. We have both had to make changes in our lives to continue living a healthy life with lupus. We have had to change our school and work dreams, we have had to stay at home when our friends were out, and we are constantly worried about if/when another flare-up may happen, and how we will cope. Yet we have done awesome things with our lives, everything we ever wanted to do!

There is no other book available at this time for teenagers and young adults with a chronic health condition like lupus. Although there are some books about lupus for children, and many more for adults, we know from our own experience that people between 13 and 30 years old are in a different category. There are many great lupus books that talk about the medical stuff, the symptoms, controlling your symptoms, medication options, etc., and we encourage you to read as many books as you like. However, we know that the medical stuff is not the only important part of living a healthy life with lupus. Jodie knows this not only from her experience of being a patient with lupus, but also from her work as a social worker within the health-care system. She is a member of a team that helps patients to deal with their emotions during/following a diagnosis, looks at their finances, considers their family's feelings, explores new career options, and connects with community resources to help with anything the patient may need. Jessica also understands that living life with lupus is not just about the medical stuff. When she was first diagnosed and began treatment, her lupus was brought under control, but it was everything else that seemed to be out of control, such as her career options, her educational commitments, her body image, her friendships, etc. When she tried to find information on those types of things, she couldn't find anything geared to young adults living with a chronic illness – that's why she teamed up with Jodie to write this book!

Why This Book?

You are living with a chronic health condition, but along with that, you are also dealing with school, trying to fit in with your friends, and choosing classes to get the job that you want. You are living with lupus and trying to develop your individuality and become independent, starting a new career and needing to prove yourself. You are living with a stressful illness, dealing with love and romantic relationships, needing to be financially stable and independent, trying to develop your self-esteem and sense of self, as well as trying to figure out how to cope with other stressful life stuff. We know that you are going through all of this, and trying to figure out how you are going to accept how lupus is changing your life, your dreams and yourself as a person, because we have been there. We decided to choose the title *Fabulupus* because we want you to know that you can still have a fabulous life with lupus. You don't have to give up on your goals or dreams. We know that your diagnosis has changed your life, but that doesn't have to be a bad thing! We hope to show you how changes that seem to be negative, like being diagnosed and living with lupus, can be positive and can help you grow as a person. Sure, some things will change – some things simply have to change in order for you to heal and succeed. You will have to be flexible and you will have to adapt to a new life, but everything that you've wanted to achieve in life is still possible. We know – we've done it. In this book, we offer lots of practical tips and tricks that we've learned along the way. Mostly, though, we want you to understand and accept that you will have to adjust parts of your life to accommodate lupus in order to reach your goals. Even with lupus, your dreams are still out there waiting for you. You can do it! We hope that this book serves as inspiration to you, and to those who are close to you.

We know that lupus affects every single aspect of your life, so we have written chapters about how to deal with lupus when it comes to: school, careers, money, relationships, spirituality, travel, healthy eating, staying active, stress, energy levels, self-esteem and style. These are all areas of your life that are very important to your coping and quality of life when living with lupus, but are not always dealt with by your medical team. We have written this book based on our experiences and the experiences of our other friends who have lupus. We hope that our trials and tribulations while trying to find what works best for us to help us live balanced lives will help you on your lupus journey.

MOST IMPORTANTLY, ALWAYS REMEMBER THAT:

We all have a different definition of quality of life;

**Knowing that you have options can help you
cope with having lupus;**

We grow through every challenge that we face in life;

The key is not being afraid to ask for help;

You can have lupus and still live life to the fullest.

RELATIONSHIPS

Family Ties

Aww, family. Can't live with them, can't live without them. Here is the unavoidable truth: your relationship with your family will change following your diagnosis, regardless of whether your diagnosis has been a long time coming versus a sudden onset, or whether you've just been diagnosed versus having been diagnosed for years. To put things into perspective, **your diagnosis can be considered an important life change that will affect your relationship with your immediate and extended family both positively and negatively for the remainder of your life** – much like other significant life events such as graduation, starting a career and marriage. With each life change, there will be some individuals in your family who will be wholly supportive, while others will challenge your ability to handle the new responsibility; some will question your motives and your credibility, while others will become overly sensitive.

To get a little more specific, if you are diagnosed while you're attending high school, your parents/guardians will of course be worried about your health, but they will also be concerned about your time off from school, the effects on your social life and self-esteem, the likelihood of you being able to complete your high school diploma and then get and hold down a job. If you are diagnosed while you're attending university/college, your parents will have similar concerns, which will extend to such things as completing your degree/ diploma and pursuing a career in your chosen field (or at all); their concerns might extend to your personal life, because of your increasing age and the likelihood that they have thought about you getting married (this will be much more obvious for those who are in a relationship at the time of diagnosis). If you are diagnosed as a young adult in the prime of your career, after having completed the necessary education, your parents/guardians will still have all the same concerns, hoping that your diagnosis will not change who you are emotionally, cognitively, educationally, and socially – and that you will be able to find a balance in managing your condition within your existing lifestyle. Of course, added frustration for parents comes from knowing that you have no control over how severe your illness will be (or become). This adds an extra dimension of complication and uncertainty, which escalates all the other worries to a new level.

All of the concerns held by your parents will likely lead to many frustrations for you because your parents may become highly protective, perhaps to a point that you may consider to be intrusive. This means that they may want to know every detail of every day, much beyond what the average teenager (or young adult) would have to share (such as how you slept, your energy throughout the day, how much hair you are losing, how much weight you are gaining/losing, your bowel movements, etc.). Your choice then becomes whether to share the complete truth, or the partial truth, or to maintain your privacy (which will likely only strengthen your parents' suspicions that you are not caring for yourself properly). This is particularly challenging for those of you who are teenagers, because you typically still live with your parents and attend doctor's appointments with their support. However, be warned, because even if you are a young adult living outside your parents' home, their worry will not lessen, and could even be heightened. Case in point: Jessica's mother still calls to ask her if she's taken her medications, even though Jessica is (at press time) 33 years old and has a child of her own! Keep in mind that the questions could be more frequent because of distance and/or lack of daily contact/observation.

So, how do you balance being a normal teenager and your parents' concerns without overstressing yourself (and potentially putting your health at risk)? Jodie found that sharing most of the truth was the best option to demonstrate that she paid attention to the important parts of her illness and their effects on her daily living. Meanwhile, she maintained some secrecy regarding unimportant details, particular aspects of discussions with psychologists and social workers that were private, as well as aspects of her relationships with friends and boyfriends. Although it was definitely annoying to have her parents reminding her to take her medication when necessary, Jodie found that the more information she kept from her parents, the more they pushed and became overprotective. Likewise, the more times Jodie demonstrated that she was responsible (and the more she shared with her parents), the more freedoms were permitted, which eventually led to even more trust from her parents.

Unfortunately, there were some other adolescents who attended the same lupus clinic as Jodie who had completely different stories. One did not have the support of her family. Her family did not understand her diagnosis and disowned her (believing she had caused her illness and feeling that it was shameful for the family), despite her responsible handling of her medical appointments, medication and daily living. This is more a reflection of her family's coping skills (or lack thereof) than of this young woman's approach, but is still worth sharing. This family's story is an extreme example of how different individuals cope with change in different ways. Although it might seem that you are the one who is going through everything, and everyone else is breathing down your neck, always remember that your parents harp on at you out of love and concern. Your parents feel responsible for your diagnosis (What did we do that caused your lupus?), they feel out of control and hurt, they are lost and scared due to the uncertainty of the condition, they are worried for your present and future, and they feel the loss associated with all they had hoped for your life and that might no longer be possible. So, when interacting with your sometimes annoying parents, always remember that things could be a whole lot worse. No matter what your situation is, all we ask is that you take a few minutes to reflect on how your parents might be feeling, consider why they are constantly barraging you with questions, and then suck it up and be thankful for the support you have (whether it be from your parents, other family members or your friends) to help get you through the crazy ride that is life; one that is further complicated by having a chronic illness.

Of course, when we speak about your family's role and their perspective on your diagnosis and future living, we cannot ignore your siblings. **Unfortunately, siblings are the most forgotten group within the health-care system,** because the medical team often does not provide guidance or support to help older and younger siblings move forward. Most of what was said about parental worries and concerns can be echoed for siblings, except their perspective is a little different. Younger siblings are likely concerned about who they will play with and who will care for them when mommy and/or daddy are not around, and can be jealous of all the attention that you are being given throughout your diagnosis, treatment and beyond. Older siblings will fondly remember you and your life goals, and will mourn the loss of any future hopes and dreams; their perspective will more closely mimic that of your parents. Teenage siblings are the most worrisome because of their already fragile emotional and hypersensitive state. Given a teenager's stage of development, they are expected to be hypersensitive to feedback from their environment, because they are trying to develop their self-identity and self-esteem, and are getting clues from their family, friends, school, activities and surroundings. Any traumatic event experienced during adolescence will likely dramatically affect their personality and future perspective on life. How much an event will influence a teenager's future is equally affected by how those around them respond, and how they are treated throughout the event, specifically how parents continue to treat them while also caring for you. Likewise, how you treat your siblings while you are sick will also have an impact on their development.

Jodie has a particularly heartbreaking example to share that perfectly illustrates this last point. Her sister was 11 years old when she was diagnosed, two years younger than Jodie. Her parents worked really hard at making special time for her sister, especially because of all the special time Jodie got to spend with her parents during hospital visits and while she was off school. When Jodie was feeling well, she also made an effort to spend time with her sister. Yet, Jodie's diagnosis definitely affected her sister's life. When her sister was interviewed for a part-time job during university, she was asked, "If you could change one thing in the world, what would you change and why?" The interviewer was expecting a response addressing poverty or global conflict, but what she got was completely unexpected. Jodie's sister got all teary-eyed and responded that she would take away Jodie's lupus because she hated to see her older sister suffer. Jodie gets teary-eyed now just thinking of her sister sitting in that interview room, crying and giving that answer!

Having a caring family is very special, but getting the right kind of care is very important. Even when someone cares about you, they can sometimes lose sight of your best interests, and get completely tangled up in trying to help you without allowing you to help yourself. They can also forget how annoying it can be to constantly have someone looking over your shoulder. If the help that is provided does not match the support that is needed, it is unlikely to be perceived as helpful or supportive by the receiver. For example, if you just need to talk to someone, and they are constantly offering to fix your problem – you get really annoyed! Equally irritating is when you just need someone to talk to, but instead people keep dropping by with food. Those who are close to you can forget to ask what you want, and what you need help with, and instead start jumping in and taking over everything. This is not only extremely annoying, but it also does not teach you to handle yourself, and your new diagnosis, while still living your life. So, how do you get the help you need, when you need it, and get rid of the unwanted offers of help when they're not needed? A fine balance is required between accepting help you do not think you need (maybe, deep-down you know you do, but are too proud to admit it) while getting the help you know you need, and still helping yourself to the maximum of your current capacity (while slowly increasing your capacity to care for yourself).

From Jodie's own experience, the trick is to allow your family to help with certain parts of your health (like driving you to and from appointments and hand-holding during painful treatments/examinations), asking for help when needed (for example helping to advocate with your teacher regarding your new needs if the teacher is not listening to you alone), and reminding your parents of what you can handle on your own (following dietary restrictions, tak-ing daily meds, etc.). These are just examples of what worked for her. Depend-ing on how your diagnosis has affected your daily abilities, which part(s) of your body is (are) affected and how much support you have from your family, you can modify this list as required. **The point is really to give your parents responsibility for some part of your care, to take responsibility for another part yourself (and to gradually build this part as you get used to things), and to ask for help when you need it.**

Friends

Dealing with friends, bringing them on board with your health issues and their associated limitations, can be similar to what you experienced with your family. Just as you have to decide to take responsibility for your health with your family, and which parts you need to ask for help with, you need to be able to acknowledge and explain these same issues with your friends. Of course, **sometimes it can be trickier to discuss your health, and its impact on your life, with your friends** than with your family. Friends can find it more difficult understand, because you are supposed to be just like them – happy and healthy! They will be confused about what you are trying to explain to them, about you being sick and being diagnosed with a chronic health condition. Aren't chronic health conditions for older people who haven't taken care of themselves throughout the years? Even more confusing is trying to explain a little-known condition like lupus, as opposed to letting your friends know you have a well-known condition like diabetes (although there are lots of misconceptions about this too!).

So, how do you decide to tell your friends about your situation? How much do you decide to share? How do you decide which friends to tell and which friends to keep your condition a secret from? These are all very personal questions, and will take a lot of pondering on your part, and possibly a discussion with someone you trust (family, close friend, doctor, social worker, etc.). Your considerations might include: How well do you know your friends? How have they treated you or others when difficult situations have come up? How do they treat your opinions on everyday things? Are they pushing for you to take their perspective? How many details you share is another personal decision. As with family, what seems to work best with friends is a balance between sharing enough details to explain your situation, while not going overboard with too many personal details.

Your friends might not understand immediately, and will push you at different stages of your relationship (and life events), but should respect your limits. Just like family, your friends might not always believe you when you say you are having a good day or a bad day, because you will likely "look" the same every day. However, your friends will quite likely be less forgiving than your family when you need to cancel at the last minute because you are suddenly not feeling well. The rest of your friends may not be feeling well either, but know that they can sleep in tomorrow and recuperate, and may not understand that you cannot recuperate in a day or two like them. From Jodie's personal experience, friends will push you a lot more than family, and interestingly, this can feel like a trap. It's a lot easier to allow your family to take care of you (and to play the sick role) and to accept being pushed by your friends (and pretending everything is fine). This imbalance can lead to a dangerous spiral of pushing too much and not pushing enough between the two parts of your life, which will likely cause you to end up sick, so it is important to address the challenge of finding the right balance in all parts of your life. Another challenge is that not only are you adjusting to the new life, but so are your friends (and family). How you interact while you are all adjusting to this new life can quickly become a pattern, and can either be helpful or harmful. Once the pattern is set, it is even harder to break, so tread carefully!

The positive side of interacting with your friends is that you will definitely find out who your true friends are. Of course, when you are in the thick of things and are really sick, losing friends is a difficult thing to accept; when you find out that you will be sick for the rest of your life, all you want is to be normal and to be surrounded by supportive friends. Just like with family members, support is only helpful if it provides you with what you need at the time. **Friends are only good if they are there for you throughout both good times and bad**, and provide you with what you need at different times of your life. Although it is challenging to accept that you may have outgrown a friendship, it is always better to be surrounded by a few really supportive individuals than a ton of people who couldn't care less about your health and happiness!

The process of losing friends is normal, and everyone goes through it, lupus or not. We will all have different friends throughout our lives, and most of our friends are usually lost or gained during major life changes. These changes typically include starting part-time work while in high school, going to college/ university, starting a career and starting a family. However, for those of us diagnosed with an illness while in adolescence or young adulthood, the most important life change that can affect our relationships can be our diagnosis.

Friendships can also change in a more positive manner. **Your diagnosis can give you an opportunity to explore new activities with your friends, activities that fit better with your new limits.** This can take some imagination at first, especially if you are in the habit of doing certain things with certain friends, but these changes can actually make your friendships stronger. They will get stronger not only because you are doing new things, and building new memories together, but because you are testing your friends' willingness to be flexible and to adjust to your new limits.

More news from the bright side is that you will likely encounter new friends along your journey, either through your hospital or through local support groups, if you feel inclined to expand your horizons and to get involved and give back (that's how Jodie & Jessica met!). Although many individuals find support groups helpful, if it's not your cup of tea and you're uncomfortable with the idea of sharing and comparing your story with others in a similar situation (getting tips on how to handle different situations and learning better health management ideas), then it's okay not to participate, but always keep the idea in the back of your mind. One day, you might want to connect with someone who is on the same life journey (and facing the same challenges) as yourself. In the meantime, don't give up on your quest for true friendship! Remind yourself of the positive aspects of your true friends as often as necessary! Remind yourself of the positive aspects of no longer having certain so-called "friends" who may have actually had a negative impact on your health and happiness.

The Dating Game

Dating is both an exciting and terrifying adventure, and having lupus can add a few more twists and turns to this journey, but having to deal with lupus doesn't mean you can't pursue romantic relationships. Having a loving partner may be just the kind of support that will really help you to cope with the uncertainty of your condition and enjoy a fulfilling life. Even if you are not looking for something serious, **dating can help you learn about yourself and what you really want out of life**. Plus, dating can be really fun! It is definitely possible to have both lupus and a fun social life, including dating possibilities.

If you are interested in dating and you feel ready to do so, meeting people is the first step. There is no shortage of places where you can meet someone. If you have a particular interest, then be sure to pursue that passion; engage in the activities that you enjoy as much as possible. By being connected with the activities that you really love, you are more likely to meet someone who shares the same interests, and you are also more likely to be your relaxed, true self. This is probably the oldest advice in the book, but it works! Another good option is to hang out in a group, as it takes a little of the pressure off and can be less stressful than one-on-one dates. The key is getting yourself out there. Even if your dating adventures only result in friendship, this is positive, because you have just widened your social network and opened yourself up to more experiences and possibilities. Plus, you probably had a good time going out, and having fun is always worthwhile. In the pursuit of a relationship, and during the process of dating, you have to be confident; try not to be afraid of rejection (easier said than done!). Having a positive attitude, an enthusiastic personality, and a bright and fun spirit is certainly attractive, and will act like a magnet in drawing others to you. And, never underestimate how happy someone else will be when you ask them out – it is flattering to know that someone likes you enough to ask you out on a date! Plus, having the courage to do this demonstrates your confidence, and shows what a catch you really are!

Meeting people can be difficult enough, but disclosing that you have lupus to a potential dating partner can be even more of a challenge. Jessica was already in a strong, long-term relationship when she was diagnosed with lupus, but she still remembers the exact moment, sitting on the outdoor steps of a building with her partner, tears streaming down her face, when she spoke the words that changed her life forever: 'I have lupus.' This was one of the hardest things she's ever had to do or say. She didn't know how he was going to react, or how he was going to feel. She didn't even know what her own feelings were! She was worried that he would reject her, even though they had already committed to each other for life, so she can only imagine how challenging it might be to tell someone whom you have only just started dating. There is already so much uncertainty in a new relationship, and adding lupus into the mix can be terrifying. This terror is augmented by the fact that lupus is such a mysterious disease that many people don't even know about. So, in addition to telling someone that you have lupus, you have to explain what lupus is, and how it affects your life! Disclosing that you have lupus to your date (and potential partner) will be an intense experience, one that will be difficult no matter what the stage of the relationship. Despite Jessica's anxiety about telling her partner, he was totally supportive. From personal experience, it is always best to tell the truth; things are so much easier when they are out in the open and explained as clearly as possible. This is not an easy task, especially because of the variability of lupus activity, but if you have lupus and you want a relationship, you will have to figure out how best to combine the two, and it all starts with being totally honest, both with yourself and with your partner.

Keep in mind that being in a relationship is not something you have to do. Certainly, it is better to be single and happy than in a relationship that is distressing and often painful. This is especially true if you are dealing with a chronic illness like lupus. Lupus management requires careful stress management, and the last thing you need is to be in a relationship that is constantly causing you stress and misery. In order to keep yourself in good health, it is very important that you are only involved in healthy and happy relationships (romantic or otherwise). This could take a little soul searching on your part, and you may need to come to terms with the fact that you should address your health first before entering into a relationship. **It is not a great idea to start looking for a partner when you are in the middle of a flare-up**. You may also need to end an existing relationship if it is hurting your health and recovery. It can be difficult to deal with the loss of a relationship, or the loss of a potential relationship you had hoped for, especially when the majority of us dream from early childhood of being in a permanent relationship. Take your time reflecting upon what will be best for you, whether you are currently experiencing a flare-up or not. Ultimately, it is about your health and happiness, not about being with a partner.

Intimacy

It is pretty much guaranteed that all of those involved in romantic relationships will face sexual challenges at some time or another. This happens in all relationships, not just those involving a partner with lupus, but there may be some specific sexual issues associated with lupus, such as the physical effects of the illness itself and the emotional consequences of dealing with this illness. Try not to be embarrassed or ashamed when you do experience difficulties. Think about it; **regardless of medical history, everyone in a relationship must deal with various challenges in relation to sexuality throughout his or her lifetime.** This is a normal part of any romantic relationship. Although this may be an uncomfortable topic, you will have to discuss intimacy issues with your partner (and likely also your doctor) in order to have a fulfilling sexual life.

Firstly, in relation to physical challenges that might limit intimacy: the hallmarks of lupus are the intense and persistent fatigue, muscle pain and joint pain. Other physical problems that can suddenly arise include rashes, pleuritis, and/or swelling. Additionally, you may experience uncomfortable side effects (such as weight gain or stomach upset) from the medications that you are taking. It is very important that you communicate with your partner and explain to them how you are feeling, and that a lack of sexual activity is caused by the lupus, not a lack of desire for or interest in your partner. If sex is not an option because of the fatigue or joint pain, perhaps you and your partner can express your affection for each other in other ways. There are unlimited ways to express your feelings for each other physically, such as hugging, kissing, petting, massage, bubble baths, etc. Consider aids such as lubrication, toys or literature. Explore the options! Be adventurous! Use your imagination! Or just relax and try again when you're feeling better.

Although it is crucial that you discuss sexual issues with your partner openly, you will also need to discuss possible medical and/or permanent solutions with your doctor. **Please be sure to talk to your doctor about any physical discomforts and how they are affecting your sex life, because this is important for your quality of life.** Before even starting a sexual relationship, it is important to discuss things with your doctor, particularly if your lupus is active and you are taking medication to help control symptoms. There are likely some precautionary measures your doctor will recommend, including delaying sexual activity due to severe lupus activity, or preferred methods of contraception (see the Family Planning section of this chapter), in addition to discussing ways of protecting yourself from sexually transmitted infections. Hopefully, you will feel comfortable talking about these issues with your doctor, but **if you are unable to talk about your sexual health, it's possible that you are not ready to enter into a sexual relationship.** We both know how awkward and potentially embarrassing these conversations can be, but please keep in mind that there is nothing to be ashamed of, your doctor is a professional who has your best interests in mind. Your love life is a key component to your health and happiness, so do your best to be honest and direct about any issues that might reduce your quality of life in this area.

Secondly, regarding emotional obstacles that may affect your sex life: the hardest part of living with a chronic health condition can be the emotional turmoil from constantly dealing with it. While coping with the physical pain and discomfort can dramatically affect your mood and fail to inspire you to feel sexy or frisky, your self-esteem may also be affected, because both the illness and the side effects of any medication you might be taking can make you feel less confident, and may lead to changes in how you perceive yourself. There may be a change in your self-image as a result of different energy levels and/or phys-ical changes in your body. Mood swings are also common, and depression is significantly more frequent in individuals with chronic health conditions than in the general population. It is especially important that you discuss these emo-tional issues with your doctor, because they are serious concerns that can affect all aspects of your life and the overall outcome of your health treatment. The emotional ramifications of lupus can take a toll on your quality of life, including your sex life. If you are feeling low, and this is affecting your physical intimacy, you need to discuss it with your partner. You will need his/her support in explor-ing other options so that your sex life remains satisfying and enjoyable. If lupus does disrupt some aspect of intimacy, then don't worry. Try to find the humor in the situation, keep the lines of communication open, talk to your doctor, be creative, be loving and know that you can always try again later (wink, wink, nudge, nudge).

Living Together with Lupus

Living with a partner will always involve challenges, and due to the un-certain nature of lupus, the challenges may be unpredictable as well! So before you decide to live with a partner, make sure you are as ready as you can be. Be sure to evaluate your reasons for wanting to move in with someone, and make sure your reasons are valid. **Many people move in together for convenience, but cohabitation can be stressful even at the best of times.** You have to con-sider how your cohabiting lifestyle will impact your lupus, and how your lupus will affect your domestic life together. You'll need to discuss all the possibilities of how moving in together might affect your relationship, and how you will need your partner's help to stay healthy. There is a lot of stuff you likely do to stay healthy when you are not with your partner, and these will all be exposed once you move in together. It is best to have this type of discussion ahead of time. If, after the discussion, you decide that you want to move in together for the right reasons, you are able to agree upon household tasks, and living with your loved one is something you are ready and prepared to do – then go ahead and take the plunge!

One of the hardest aspects of living with someone is the actual maintenance of your home, and so this topic must be part of your pre-moving-in discussion. When you live with someone, you have to negotiate on everything, including who is doing what part of the home maintenance. Fair and equitable division of labor is tough to plan and even tougher to pull off, and it is even harder when you have an illness like lupus, because it may strike at any time, and you may be temporarily unable to complete your share of the household chores due to fatigue, pain or the side effects of your medication. This is not the end of the world, though, and you should discuss the options with your partner before the situation arises. These might include ignoring certain tasks until you feel better, changing roles and doing lighter tasks while your partner tackles the heavier items, or calling on friends and family for help. For example, when Jessica is not feeling all that great, her husband will do the laundry, but Jessica will fold the clothes while watching TV and relaxing. Be creative, and use tools and/or technology to help you out. Overall, though, the most important thing is that you and your partner remain flexible, as you may need to change your priorities and tasks whenever you experience a flare-up, and each flare-up can manifest differently. **Always remember that your health is way more important than a few dirty dishes!**

When you are living with someone, they are also living with your lupus, and they are likely to react in similar ways to your family and friends, as discussed earlier. It is important to keep communicating with your partner, letting them know how you are doing, both mentally and physically, so that they're not always worrying about you. Make sure that they have a support system of their own, too. This is especially important if you become very sick, and they become your caregiver. Please be sure to appreciate your partner, and show your appreciation with both words and actions, bearing in mind that they need to be kept in the loop at all times so that they can plan their life and prepare for different scenarios with you. While living with the one you love is a joyful experience, the same may not necessarily be said of living with your lupus; however, this challenge can serve to bring you closer together, and make you focus on the really important things in your life together.

Tips for a Zen Wedding

Deciding to get married is a major life decision, one that is both wonderful and stressful, just like deciding on the type of wedding that you and your partner would like to have. This is true for every couple, but having lupus adds a new dimension, because you need to do your best to keep yourself healthy during what can potentially be a particularly demanding time in your life. We have both been 'lupus brides,' and can attest that while our weddings were perfectly lovely, the entire process was certainly not perfect! What was most important during the wedding preparations was that we both managed to stay healthy and flare-up-free, which made the big day so wonderful! Here are few 'Dos' and 'Don'ts' that we want to share with you based on our experiences:

Don't be bullied into doing what well-meaning relatives or friends want, and end up with a wedding that you didn't choose.

Don't ignore your health. You (and your health) are more important than any wedding.

Don't become obsessed about every little detail. No wedding is absolutely perfect. Remember to bask in the glow of your wedding day – this will (likely) only happen once!

Don't feel compelled to do every single thing yourself. Delegate some tasks to your partner, friends, family, wedding planner/site coordinator, or pay someone else to help.

Don't get too stressed out, because everything will turn out great.

Don't be obsessed with having a "perfect" body or a flawless face on your wedding day. Yes, you will be photographed on your wedding day, and you want your pictures to look great. However, you and your pictures don't need to be "perfect." Focus on your health, and don't be self-conscious if your body has changed. Be proud that you are conquering a major illness. Remember that on your wedding day, you are the most beautiful person in the world.

Don't try for a perfect wedding; instead, aim for a wedding that you will love.

Do recognize that there will be many elements of your wedding that you will not be able to control. So, try to relax and enjoy the experience.

Do consider wedding options such as a destination wedding, a small wedding, a small reception at a restaurant, a cocktail-style reception, or other creative choices.

Do have the type of wedding that is best for you and your partner.

Do be organized. Use tools such as lists, spreadsheets and the Internet.

Do select a comfortable and forgiving dress (in case your body does change) and choose great makeup (and/or a makeup artist) to help you feel your best!

Do your best to respect your financial situation.

Do take good care of yourself while you plan your wedding; make sure to eat well, get lots of sleep, stay active and stay relaxed.

Do vow to cherish yourself, honor your body and respect your limits while planning your wedding.

Family Planning

Having children is a huge decision that will affect every aspect of your life, so it cannot be taken lightly. This is one commitment that you will definitely need to involve two other people in, namely your partner and your doctor, and one that ideally you should also discuss with many other people, in particular your family and trusted friends. However, please be aware that, ultimately, family planning decisions are mainly yours and your partner's. You need to do what is right for you, your life and your lupus.

When you have lupus and you are considering having children, there can be some heavy emotional things to deal with. Many of these emotions can be very negative. However, it's normal to feel ambivalent about wanting a child, so don't feel bad if you're unsure about having kids. Having lupus is hard, and having kids when you have lupus might be incredibly difficult. You may feel scared, worried or understandably nervous. You might even feel angry that you have to worry about certain things that others might just take for granted. When Jessica was thinking about having kids, she felt guilty that she might "short change" her children because her illness might impact them. It's likely that you will experience some difficult feelings about having kids, but know that this is entirely normal. Many people feel the same way at some point, even those without lupus. If you feel that the emotions are too difficult to process, please talk to your partner, a family member or a trusted friend, or even consider talking to your doctor and/or a therapist. Family planning is a big decision that will change several aspects of your life, so please make sure you take care of your feelings and obtain the support that you need.

There are many factors involved in family planning, such as deciding on the right age to have children, how your career/education fits in, how your finances will be affected, etc. These are issues that almost all other couples face. However, when you have lupus, you have to think about other factors, such as the status of your illness, your physical capacities, and your energy levels. As a result, there are many additional questions and concerns. One of the more difficult aspects of family planning when you have lupus is that both the condition and the medication that is prescribed to help you deal with it can sometimes affect your fertility. That is why it is imperative that you discuss these issues with your doctor throughout your family planning process. At the same time, please don't stress about fertility to the point of constant anxiety. Almost all couples, regardless of medical history, have to deal with fertility issues, and there are always options, especially in this day and age with all of the ongoing scientific advances and improvements in medical technology. And don't forget about adoption: there are a lot of children around the world who need loving parents. But, once again, you need to do what is best for you, your partner, your health and your lifestyle.

Of course, becoming a parent warrants discussion regarding not only the physical capacity to become pregnant (or fertilize an egg, in the case of males with lupus), but also regarding whether you can stay healthy, both during your pregnancy and while raising a child. Does your partner have a secure job, so that you can stay home with the child(ren)? Or is your current career flexible enough to accommodate children and lupus? Should you consider a different career? Or, would your health be safer, and your talents be better used, if you volunteered with children in the community, and/or spoiled other children in your life (those of friends and family)? The discussions surrounding family planning are endless, and the possibilities will change with every change in your health status, so you need to keep talking with both your partner and your doctor.

When Jodie was diagnosed at age 13 years, she was suddenly thrust into discussing family planning with her doctors. Knowing whether she wanted children or not affected which medication options were available to treat her lupus symptoms. Imagine being just 13 years old and having to decide whether or not you want to have children some day! Understandably, Jodie's thoughts about wanting children changed over the years, and so it was important that she continued to communicate these changes to her doctor. In June 2008, when Jodie got engaged, her doctor immediately reevaluated the type and dosage of medication that she was taking with the hope of giving Jodie and her husband the option of trying to become pregnant in a few years. Once again, even though they weren't even married yet, they were already planning for children. When you have a chronic condition, family planning involves a lot of discussions and planning procedures. The most important thing is to keep yourself healthy and happy, and to do the things that will bring you peace and joy.

Your relationships with your family (present and future) and friends (present and future) will be impacted by your diagnosis to varying degrees, but always remember all relationships are fluid, and change over time. Sometimes they are easy and fun, and sometimes they are challenging and stressful. Sometimes you will need to step up the level of communication to keep moving forward with the relationship, and sometimes you will need to let some relationships go. It's not easy, but having great relationships in your life is key to your happiness, your success and your ability to cope with your illness. Having fabulous people in your life will just make you even more fabulous than you already are!

SCHOOL & EDUCATION

Plan Your Path

Most young people have to juggle heavy textbooks, heavy course loads, and heavy extracurricular commitments, but we also have to juggle lupus. Most young people ask themselves, "What am I going to do with my life?" Those of us who are diagnosed with lupus have to ask ourselves, "What am I going to do with my life *now that I have lupus*?"

Many people with lupus are diagnosed while they are still in school. Finishing your current school program while having lupus is hard enough, but what happens after you graduate? Having lupus may have a dramatic impact not only on your current schooling, but also on any future educational plans. For those who have to swallow a lot of pills, this may be the toughest pill of all to swallow. Many of us have big goals and even bigger dreams, and these ambitions may require further schooling or training. Because managing both school and lupus is already challenging, the thought of even *more* school may seem unappealing, daunting, or even downright impossible.

What is also unappealing, daunting, and seemingly impossible is the fact that you will likely need to accept that lupus will affect both your short- and long-term goals. There may be periods of sadness or feelings of hopelessness when you are thinking about your future education. It's okay to feel confused and irritated at your situation. Gradually, accepting that lupus may affect your school plans will set in, but this process toward acceptance is not easy, and usually doesn't happen immediately. Accepting that lupus will affect your education is especially hard when it seems like your friends have no cares in the world, and are simply looking forward to graduating and going on to bigger and better things. It's okay to grieve; lupus is a major life-changing illness. But, also realize that *you too* will be moving on to bigger and better things. You can complete your schooling, and you can pursue even more education if you want to. Sure, things might be a little different than you expected, but that's okay. Actually, **having a condition like lupus will strongly motivate you to figure out what you truly love to do and what you truly want to accomplish in life.** If you are currently in school, it is actually a great place to start thinking about what really interests you and in what direction you want to go. Most schools have plenty of resources, so take advantage of guidance counselors and teachers. Schools also offer a variety of courses and clubs. Start paying attention to what you really enjoy and what you excel at. Now is the time to start looking at all of the options, to do research, and to ask questions. Find what you love to do! Although having lupus was certainly not part of the path you had previously planned, your lupus might steer you in directions that you would have never previously considered, and this new path can be incredible!

Lupus + School = Success!

Initially, it may seem that lupus hinders our ability to cope with school and the stress of school hinders our ability to cope with lupus. Yet, education is a major weapon in the fight to have a happy and productive life while having lupus. The unpredictability of lupus is by far the biggest hurdle to deal with when it comes to choosing your courses for the next semester, or choosing the right educational program, or deciding on anything to do with your future. You have no idea when the next flare-up will strike, nor can you forecast the size or severity of each flare-up. Because it is really hard to know what your state of health will be in a few months, let alone in a few years, it may seem impossible to plan your future. Sometimes it may be so frustrating that there seems little point in even bothering to try to come up with a strategy for your life. But there is hope – and that hope is education.

Education is so powerful, because it gives you options. Having access to a number of different options is incredibly valuable and reassuring, because it gives you flexibility throughout your life. When you have more options, you can choose any number of different paths at any point in your lupus journey. **Knowing that you have options can help you cope with having lupus.** Education can open many different doors for you, especially because being diagnosed with lupus can feel like every door is being slammed shut. If at any time in your life you need to change your career or lifestyle (for whatever reason), you will be able to make these transitions much easier if you have a variety of skills.

Jessica was diagnosed while she was working on her master's degree in biology, and because of her lupus (in addition to other factors), she decided to pursue a career rather than continuing her studies, so while she was completing her research project for her master's degree, she made sure to focus on the skills involved in planning experiments and coordinating projects. After completing her studies, she became a study coordinator organizing truly beneficial (and at the same time really interesting) cancer research initiatives. She was able to transition into a better option for herself because she had a solid education and because she really maximized her skill set and put it to good use. So yes, having lupus may change your planned course for your life. It will continue to influence practically every decision you make throughout your life, and as a result you must remain flexible, and prepared to choose new routes.

However, for many people with lupus, the struggle to stay in school is a real concern, so it is important to focus on the benefits of education and training. The most important thing is to at least complete high school. Having a high school diploma will give you many options that might not have otherwise been available. After finishing high school, you can decide if more schooling is right for you, your future plans, and your continued health. We recognize that not everyone's health will permit him or her to continue his or her education. However, do not despair, there are many great advantages from being involved in volunteering that can help you in a future career. We talk more about volunteering later in this chapter.

There are plenty of other really cool benefits from education: **education is an incredibly empowering experience, because in school you are constantly faced with problems that enable you to gain confidence as you solve each and every one of them.** School can also be a fun place to be, as there are tons of activities and social events connected to school programs. School is a place where you meet some cool people and make great friends. School expands your social network, and having supportive friends can really help you cope with your illness. School can also provide a professional network, and these key contacts may prove to be invaluable when you are looking for a job or need career guidance. Keep in mind that school is more than just facts and figures: you also learn and hone transferable life skills, such as time management and organization. Lupus will continue to throw curve balls at you throughout your life, and it's a lot easier to manage if you have some tricks up your sleeve. So keep learning and keep growing! Knowledge is power, and lupus can never take that away from you.

School Daze

Jessica was a happy-go-lucky graduate student doing fun and exciting biology research, but halfway through her master's she was diagnosed with lupus. Initially, she focused on getting better and adjusting to a new life of daily medications and seemingly constant medical appointments, but once she fell into the groove of being a 'lupus patient,' she had to face another test; how was she going to cope with being a 'lupus student'? This is a question that all young lupus patients face. Most people with lupus are diagnosed when they are teenagers or young adults, and for the most part while they are still in school. Despite dealing with this new illness, many students continue on and complete their schooling. Furthermore, many young people with lupus pursue additional education through graduate-level studies or extra degrees/certificates. Such accomplishments are incredibly admirable, and are not without their challenges.

Although there are so many benefits to school, it is difficult to deal with the many problems associated with lupus while trying to attend classes. Depending on the nature of your illness, you might have to face issues that may slow down learning, such as intense fatigue and/or pain, multiple medical appointments, and even hospitalizations. If lupus is interfering with your schooling, you need to have options. There is no universal solution for these problems, as each person with lupus has different issues.

However, there are some common strategies that we can all use.

PLAN ahead. Think of any potential problems, both big and small, that may occur, and write them down if that helps to keep you organized. (See the sample list below). Predicting the tough issues that you may face can be discouraging and de-motivating, but there are options available for you! It is always better to anticipate problems and plan ahead than to be caught off-guard.

Be PROACTIVE. With your list in mind, do your research to see what support is available. Talk to people and seek the resources that you may require.

Stay ORGANIZED. Use a calendar and day planner (electronic or paper); keep them updated with due dates for assignments, tests, and medical appointments. Keep your notes and binders organized and easily accessible.

Set PRIORITIES. Make frequent checklists so that you can focus on what needs to get done right away. Be realistic about timelines and workflow. If you need help or more time, it is always best to let your teachers/instructors know well in advance. Don't do too many extracurricular activities, and cut down on them if they become too overwhelming. Always remember that your health is your number-one priority.

Keep in mind that it will take you a while to adjust to managing both school and lupus, so take your time to figure out what works best for you. **Don't get discouraged; some strategies will work right away and some will take more time to develop.** If you find that attending school full-time is too difficult, there are many alternative routes to achieving your goals. Depending on the type of schooling that you are doing, there are all kinds of options such as going to school part-time, taking distance/correspondence courses, or doing online courses. You may also need to consider why you are interested in pursuing a particular field (for example, do you like health care because you want to work with people, or because you want to find a cure for a disease?). This could lead you to reconsider what type of education is necessary for you to reach your goal (for example, university versus college; work experience versus educational experience). If your health needs are not at all compatible with school, then you should re-prioritize to focus solely on your health. There are plenty of options that will enable you to continue learning outside of traditional, structured educational settings. Consult with your doctor; talk to your teachers and family. Don't worry about the time factor: what is most important is that you are healthy!

Sample List of Potential "School" Problems and Solutions:

Potential Problems	Potential Solutions
Missing class because of illness	Arrange for the teacher/instructor or a classmate to pass on notes to keep you updated Try to do as much of the assigned readings and/or read the teacher's handouts while you are resting at home or in hospital
Class schedule is too intense and full	Discuss with your instructor or coordinator to see what classes can be done at a later time, or perhaps you can do a special assignment instead of taking one of the courses
Difficulty taking notes because of joint pain	Arrange for a note-taker (either through disability services or by asking the instructor)
Large research project (for graduate thesis)	Discuss with your supervisor and see if project can be downsized and still get results, or perhaps other people can help Discuss and set a reasonable and flexible time frame to work on and complete a project

Keep in mind that each problem may have a different solution depending on the level of education, so keep updating this list while you transition through different schools and programs!

Financing Your Education

Scholarships

In today's world, education is an absolute necessity for finding employment and having a paycheck to meet your daily needs; unfortunately it is a very expensive necessity. The financial implications of completing your education while having a chronic health condition like lupus continue to increase. The increased cost of education is related not only to taking longer (likely) to complete your degree, but also to health-related costs (which do not disappear while someone is a student). However, there is light at the end of the tunnel! Having a chronic health condition, having a goal of achieving a particular career, and having demonstrated a dedication to achieving your goal in spite of your health condition all combine to increase your chances of receiving a scholarship or bursary to offset the costs of your educational pursuits.

More specifically, there are numerous scholarships dedicated to individuals with particular conditions – such as blindness, missing limbs, brain injury, and cancer – as well as to individuals with chronic health conditions in general. The key to receiving these scholarships is to demonstrate (through your written application) the negative effects of your condition on your day-to-day living, including student life. However, you must also demonstrate your dedication to completing your education in spite of your condition, how your condition has increased your determination to achieve your goal, and how having a chronic condition will influence your career once you are working in your chosen field.

Likewise, there are scholarships dedicated to individuals studying certain disciplines, such as business/commerce, sociology, and physics. Sometimes these types of scholarships are offered to applicants who have a chronic health condition, are of a specific gender, or can show financial need. For example, to encourage females to study in nontraditional fields like mathematics and the sciences, there are often scholarships dedicated to female applicants. Likewise, there is a pull for individuals with chronic health conditions to study in the fields of social sciences and arts.

Although applying for scholarships might seem really scary, and too much hard work, the end result – *free money* – is always worth the effort. It takes a little time management, and some practice writing application letters, but it will enhance your educational experience and reduce the stress that we all have in relation to the ever-rising cost of studying beyond high school. Be sure to have someone go over your application, not only for general editing purposes, but also to assess whether your application is clear and convincing. Once you have completed a couple of applications, you will be able to reuse a lot of the same information for subsequent scholarship applications.

So the big question now is: how do you find out about scholarships that are available to you? If you are in high school and preparing to attend university, you can start by talking to your guidance counselor, checking with the school you have applied to enter, and searching on the Internet. There are also books published annually that list the various organizations offering scholarships, the requirements, and the application deadlines. If you are at college or university, you can talk to your financial aid office, the office for students with disabilities, and the career center, you can search on the Internet, and once again, you can search the annual books listing the various scholarships that are available. In addition, ask your family if their place of employment (or the place where they volunteer) offers special scholarships. It is often surprising to learn which organizations offer scholarships, and their requirements, so search far and wide, and apply for as many as possible.

Although education is getting more and more expensive, consider it an investment in your future. Sometimes it can be frightening to think of how much it will cost for you to complete your education, but once you have achieved your goal, and are working in a field you enjoy, you will gradually be able to repay your student loans. Decreasing the amount that you will need to repay is a no-brainer, but it will only happen if you receive scholarships or bursaries....and guess what? **There are thousands of dollars' worth of scholarships that are not claimed each year simply because no one bothered to apply**! Feeling any more motivated to take the time to write a few scholarship applications now?

Borrowing money

Although there is money available to almost all those who apply for scholarships, and certain individuals will be fortunate enough to have their parents/guardians pay for their education, the reality is that the majority of us will need to pay for our education ourselves. We can meet some of the costs with money saved during the summer and (possibly) from working part-time while attending school, but typically students do not make enough from these sources to be able to pay for their entire year. So, unfortunately, we are left with no choice but to borrow money. The most common place to borrow money is through a government student loan program, but generally, during your first five years of post-secondary education, the government takes your parents' income into consideration. This means that if your parents make a lot of money, you will not be able to borrow as much, because the government assumes that if your parents are making a certain amount of money, they should be contributing to your education (even if this is not the reality, for any number of reasons). However, after the first five years of post-secondary education, the government considers students to be independent, which means you can borrow more money because your parents' income and (assumed) contribution to your education is no longer considered. To obtain a government loan, you need to apply online during the late spring or early summer prior to beginning your studies in September. One benefit of taking out a government loan is that when it comes time to repay the loan, any interest that you pay can be claimed on your taxes. That might not mean much right now, but when you're working and earning a paycheck, it can make a big difference. Another benefit of government loans for individuals with lupus and other conditions and disabilities is that once a loan has been approved, the recipient will receive an additional amount to help cover any disability-related costs. To receive this additional amount, you need to talk to the disability office at your institution, which then needs to communicate to the government to confirm that you are enrolled as a student with a disability.

There are several other options for those who either do not qualify for a government loan or simply decide to borrow money from somewhere else. The main alternative is to establish a line of credit at the bank. Typically, you will need a parent to co-sign for this loan. Although bank loans usually have slightly lower interest rates than government loans, you cannot claim any interest from your bank loan on your taxes. Another option is borrowing from your family or friends. Borrowing money from family/friends typically means that you do not have to pay any interest, but can sometimes cause friction in the relationship.

Of course, you should also consider ways to reduce the cost of completing your education, like living at home with your parents instead of moving away, taking longer to complete your education so that you can work while going to school, and comparing the cost of attending the various schools you are interested in. For example, in Canada, those living in the province of Quebec pay one-third of the tuition fees of other Canadians to attend university within the province, and the cost of living in Montreal, Quebec is lower than in many other cities across Canada.

Educational support for success

No matter where you live, where you borrow money from, or where you manage to obtain free money, we all need support to successfully complete our education to the best of our abilities. We need to put support systems into place to reduce the effects of our health condition on our ability to meet scholarly expectations. At high school, we can do this by meeting with our guidance counselor. Typically, this is the person who would speak with your teachers about the special accommodations you need to succeed. At college or university, the office for students with disabilities would typically assist with the necessary accommodations. **Accommodations that most students with chronic health conditions receive include extra time on assignments (as needed), extra time to complete exams, writing exams in a private room, and access to special technology to complete exams/assignments.** But, these are just examples – different schools have different options, so be sure to ask!

Before you start to receive accommodations, a school will usually ask for a meeting with you and your family (especially at high school), during which they will discuss your condition and what types of accommodations you think you will need to successfully complete your school year. They will also typically ask for a letter from your doctor outlining how your condition affects your ability to complete your education. At most schools, once you are registered as a student with a health condition, you are able to take fewer courses without being penalized. Most students (at high school or university) need to take 4–5 classes per semester to be considered full-time (this amount will differ at high school depending on whether your school uses the semester or non-semester format), however, students registered with a disability only need to take 3 classes per semester to be considered full-time at most institutions. A student needs to be registered full-time to benefit from most student services (sports complex, health services, city transport passes…in addition to loans and scholarships). Taking fewer courses can also help you manage the stress of being a student and meeting your student responsibilities, while staying healthy.

Once you are registered as a student with a disability, you need to stay in regular contact with your guidance counselor (or the personnel at the college/university office for students with disabilities) throughout the remainder of your studies. They will make all the special arrangements that you need when it comes time for you to write exams, and will make sure that you are getting the accommodations you need in each of your classes (this is particularly handy if certain professors prove difficult to deal with). At college/university, they can also communicate with your academic advisor to make a special education plan for you to complete your degree in your own time (this role is also part of the guidance counselor's tasks at high school). As you progress in your studies, your contact person can adjust your accommodations as needed if, for example, your condition worsens.

Always be aware that you have many options with respect to proper accommodations and financial support (which really can reduce the stress of being a student with a disability!). Hopefully, with all of this information in mind, you are feeling even more motivated to go forth and attain all your educational goals.

Back to School

It is said that our generation can expect to have at least five different careers throughout our lifetime – which quite logically leads to the conclusion that most of us will return to school in our later years to either boost our current level of education or to completely change fields. Some of us might return to school several times and maintain a regular pattern of periods of employment mixed with periods of education throughout our entire adulthood. For those of us with a chronic health condition, returning to school could also mean returning to complete our high school diploma. Some of us will suffer from lupus so severely throughout our adolescence that we might have to stop attending regular high school. No matter the reason, returning to school is a huge consideration, a difficult decision, and one that presents many challenges. **Any life change, no matter how positive, can be very stressful...and those with chronic health conditions, like lupus, need to do their best to reduce their levels of stress.** Learning to accept change, how to ask for help, and to move forward positively are key skills to continue to live well with your lupus.

One obvious challenge will be adjusting to a new schedule while ensuring that we maintain our health and take care of other life responsibilities. Typically, attending college/university offers a more flexible schedule than working full-time, and this more flexible schedule is often also an option for those returning to complete high school. However, with increased flexibility comes the need for increased organization; you will need to learn to manage your own time. For example, you may only have classes for three hours a day, and may not have any assignments to hand in for a couple of weeks, but in a few weeks you will have to submit two research papers and write one exam. You will need to organize your time and complete those assignments now, to give you time to study closer to the date of your exam. This type of organization is different than that required when working full-time, which (for most of us) generally means meeting daily/weekly deadlines. Likewise, (usually) when you're working, you know that when you leave your office at the end of the day, and prior to weekends, you don't need to worry about work for a while, whereas once you return home from school, even if it's only three hours of classes daily, you will need to continue to work in order to stay on top of assignments and exams.

When returning to school, there is likely also anxiety related to potential changes in how school is taught and how to study. Not too long ago online learning was not a common option, and students did not bring their laptops to class for the purpose of taking notes. Now the online learning community is an integral part of many campuses and learning institutions, which can be a great option for those with lupus. Therefore, when returning to school, it is best to fully educate yourself regarding the options available at your chosen institution. This might mean meeting with the academic advisor, the career advisor, and the disability advisor to ensure that all your needs are met and increase your chance of success in a new world.

Things to consider when returning to school include your reasons for returning, what you hope to accomplish, and both your place and program of study. Always make sure to take care of yourself in the process! However, the most important thing is to enjoy the experience of learning!

Education Where You Least Expect It

Lifelong learning is imperative to surviving in today's job market. Furthermore, having an expanded set of skills can help you move forward if you experience any lupus-based setbacks. The best news is that there are plenty of opportunities to expand your skills, both inside and outside of standard education programs, and without adding too much to your already busy schedule. **It**

is never too early or too late to adopt a lifelong learning attitude!

Ongoing education

There are plenty of opportunities within standard educational settings to boost your skills within your chosen field, or to add new skills outside of your present field of employment, without returning to school full-time. Many colleges and universities offer weekend or evening courses to fulfill diploma and certificate programs. These can be taken to deepen your understanding of a particular aspect of your current program of study or your current job, or it could be to learn something completely new. For example, even though Jodie has earned her master's degree in social work and has learned essential counseling skills, she could complete a weekend certificate to specialize in a particular therapeutic technique, or to understand the differences between counseling teenagers and counseling the elderly.

Another way of learning outside of traditional educational settings is attending workshops and conferences. Typically, people within the same profession, who work with a similar population, or who are interested in the same topic area attend these types of events. They are a great way to learn a few new things, and to meet others who are "into" the same things as you. One of the great advantages of lifelong learning is the benefit of networking – maintaining established links and building new connections. **Employers are invariably attracted to individuals who are dedicated to improving their skill set – both when hiring and when it comes time for promotion**. Plus, any expenses associated with lifelong learning activities can usually be claimed on your taxes as educational or employment-related expenses. There are many benefits in addition to learning something new!

Although you might hear about workshops and conferences through your personal networks, they are also typically advertised at your workplace or at your school. This ensures that individuals who are studying or working in a particular field are made aware of any relevant workshops and conferences. There are also plenty of other opportunities at work and at school to boost your skills. At work, there are opportunities to join committees, or to shadow someone doing a slightly different job, and there are sometimes professional development activities offered on-site that target specific areas that the managerial or administrative team feel are important to the majority of employees. Conferences, workshops, and professional development opportunities are great for those lacking the time or money to commit to formal education.

Similar activities are also available at school. For example, you can join committees, or you can become a mentor or mentee (helping younger students, or learning from someone already working in your desired field, respectively). Some high schools and universities even offer an opportunity for high school students to become a college/university student for a day or a week.

Volunteering

In addition to the "free" training opportunities listed above, we believe that there is also a lot of merit in volunteering. You may choose to volunteer in a sector that is completely different from your current place of employment to expand your skills, to enjoy a change of pace, or simply to feel that you are contributing to humankind. You may also choose to volunteer to expand your range of work-related skills, to meet new people with a common interest, and/or to boost your social links with others who work in your field. Volunteer connections can often lead to either educational opportunities or future employment, either within the agency where you are volunteering or through the connections you make by volunteering. Additional benefits from volunteering are well documented. Those who volunteer have been found to be happier with their lives, to have higher self-esteem, and to have reduced overall life stress (see the references listed at the end of this chapter). Apparently, **no matter how busy your schedule, if you manage to fit in some volunteering, your health will benefit, in addition to your skills.**

So don't let your lupus stop you from attaining a wide variety of skills. As you can see, there are many opportunities available for you to expand your skill set, both professionally and personally, and almost all of them can be undertaken within the framework of your condition. You don't need to do every-thing all at once. Take your time, and do what you really want to do – when you can do it. Sure, you may need to be more creative and resourceful (which are key skills themselves!), but the effort will certainly be worth it.

References

Hamilton, S. & Fenzel, M. (1988). *The impact of volunteer experience on adolescent social development: Evidence of program effects*, Journal of Adolescent Research, 65(70).

Johns Hopkins Medicine. (2004). Gaining health while giving back, Press Release. Available at www.hopkinsmedicine.org/Press_releases/2004/04_06_04.html

Corporation for National and Community Services. (2007). *The health benefits of volunteering: A review of recent research.* Available at www.nationalservice.gov/pdf/07_0506_hbr.pdf

Volunteer Canada. (2011). *Why volunteer? Benefits to the community – and you.* Available at www.volunteer50plus.ca/benefits.php

Resources

National Student Loan Services
http://www.canlearn.ca/eng/index.shtml

CAREERS & EMPLOYMENT

Lupus@Work

Although there are many benefits from having a job (paycheck, woo-hoo!), the challenges that lupus presents simply cannot be ignored. Your concerns about having to balance both your work life and lupus life are entirely reasonable, and should not be trivialized. You will need to develop some strategies to balance a satisfying job and a manageable illness, bearing in mind that it may take some time to adjust to a new working environment, but work is exactly that: work, and sometimes it can get a little crazy.

The cornerstone of any happy and functional life is equilibrium. Establishing and maintaining a good work–health–life balance with your specific career and your particular lupus condition is especially important given that managing the symptoms of lupus requires managing your stress levels. Whenever you are starting new job, it's a good idea to identify what might be stressful so that you can proactively figure out some solutions.

As you progress along your career path, keep an eye out for both the stressful elements associated with your job, as well as those related to your home life, so that you can develop appropriate coping skills. The best general tip we can give to prevent you from becoming overly stressed at work is to be organized: be sure to keep your calendar updated, create (and update) "to-do" lists so that you can focus on daily and weekly priorities, and be realistic about timelines and workflows. **However, the most important skill to learn and implement is to say "No" and to be willing to acknowledge when you are becoming overloaded before your health becomes affected.** Be honest with your employer, your co-workers, and yourself if your workload becomes too overwhelming as they can always find ways of accommodating the situation. Some solutions may be simpler than you thought! It may seem daunting to ask for more time if you have just started in a new position, but that is precisely the reason why you need to be cut some slack: you are new, and still learning the ropes. Alternatively, if you suddenly find yourself overwhelmed, even if you've been in the position for a while, your employer may be more willing to show some flexibility because you have already proven yourself. It's a win–win situation! The key is communicating your concerns before the situation gets out of control, having some sort of contingency plan, and some creative, resourceful ideas. Most importantly, keep a close eye on your health. You can achieve a satisfying and productive life, it just takes a little bit of monitoring, organization, and creativity.

If you are constantly feeling miserable about your job, and are struggling to cope with the demands, then perhaps you need to reassess your priorities in life. Consult your doctor to determine the status of your health. In addition, think about consulting with financial planners and educational counselors to assess the various options that are open to you. The right job for you is out there somewhere, so don't get discouraged. Goals can always be achieved when you feel well enough to take them on!

Embarking on Your Career Path

Most of us start to think seriously about what we want to do with our lives while we are completing high school. We get inspiration by thinking about which courses we have enjoyed throughout high school, which courses we have excelled at, and what other aspects of our lives inspire us, as well as thinking about the individuals we admire and their careers. We might also reflect deeply upon personal experiences, such as being diagnosed with a chronic medical condition. Some of us will also seek guidance from our family and friends, while others will get ideas from our teachers, or our school's career counselors. These are all valid methods of narrowing the number of career options, and their effectiveness is a truly based on the individual. However, based upon our personal experiences, we recommend using a combination of these strategies. For example, Jodie based her career decision upon her deeply personal experience of being diagnosed with a chronic health condition as a young teenager. This sparked her interest in becoming an adolescent counselor. Through discussions with her high school's career counselor, and completion of personality-career matching questionnaires, they discovered that this was an ideal career for her personality strengths and weaknesses. Thereafter, Jodie pursued a bachelor's degree in psychology, which led to bachelor's and master's degrees in social work – the career that she currently occupies (and enjoys!).

Finding a balance between achieving your dream career and respecting the limits imposed by your health can be quite challenging. We all have high hopes and big dreams in relation to what we would like to do with our lives, what we would like to contribute to the world, and what legacy we would like to leave behind, as well as how much we would like to earn. However, when we have a chronic health condition, finding a balance between our dream job and what we can physically accomplish – while staying healthy – is even more challenging. **Some of us are more accepting of our limits, while others have to challenge their limits to help define the exact boundaries.** As with other aspects of our lives, we need to constantly remind ourselves of all the blessings in our lives, and to accept what we cannot change.

Nowadays, we have access to many career options that can be both practical and fulfilling, and can lead to a productive and satisfying life. Despite what you may think, having lupus does not need to be an all-or-nothing situation. It is now possible to have both lupus and a very (emotionally and financially) gratifying career, although this requires a few important qualities. Among these qualities are acceptance, some soul-searching, some creativity and flexibility, and a positive attitude.

Lupus will always play a big role in your life, so, you have to ask yourself: how can I have lupus and yet still have the life I want? One of the first and most difficult things to do is to accept that lupus will factor into your career choices. The degree to which lupus may interfere with future or current career goals will depend on the stage in your life you were at when you were diagnosed and the severity of your illness. Unfortunately, you may have to mourn the loss of previous career ambitions that may no longer be sustainable. You may even have to let go of the vision of who you thought you would be and reshape your goals and your definition of yourself. It's okay to feel sad, mad, cheated, and confused. Anyone who has been diagnosed with lupus (or any other chronic illness) has probably faced the same issues, so if you're feeling really lonely, angry, or lost, this is entirely normal. Eventually, you will learn to process all of these feelings; you will keep going, in one way or another, with your life, as you transition through various life opportunities. **If you need help working through your feelings and how they are affecting your life, talk to someone**. Although your feelings are normal, it can take time to adjust to the idea of changing your career path, or to the idea of taking advantage of new opportunities in your life.

The most important thing to consider is that changes in your career don't necessarily have to be negative. In fact, these changes may even lead to a better career and improved health. Change can be very frustrating to accept, but can guide you to a very happy place. Although it may seem you are being forced to consider different career options to better manage your health, in the end you will actually be better off than some of your healthy peers who were not given the opportunity to thoughtfully reflect on and choose their best possible future. So, when the tough choices are banging on your door, demanding your attention, **remember that there can always be something positive that comes from negative life circumstances**. For example, someone interested in helping youth might find counseling too stressful, and might turn to conducting research about youth instead. Likewise, someone interested in becoming a high-profile travel journalist might find the position too taxing on their physical health, and may become a writer for a local journal or a freelance contributor to multiple columns instead. Choosing a career that offers options and/or less stress will be better for your health, and might open up a whole new world of possibilities at the same time.

Though it's not easy, this soul-searching process can ultimately be an uplifting experience, and the resulting outcomes can bring you joy, fulfillment, and better health. It may even result in a better career, with better pay, more prestige, and more fulfillment. You now have the opportunity to really find out who you are and what your values are; and remember, you have the power to decide which option is best for you. You will have to ask yourself deep and personal questions, such as "What am I passionate about?" and "What do I value?" There are also practical questions to consider based on your illness, such as "What are my ideal working conditions?" For more key questions, see the following list.

Of course, the answers to these types of questions are as varied as the career possibilities that are out there for you. Because lupus manifests itself differently in each individual, it follows that every career journey will also be different. **Don't feel that you have to do what everyone else is doing or what people expect of you.** This is your life. Find out what you can and want to do. No one said it would be simple. Finding your purpose in life isn't supposed to be easy! Seek help. There are many resources available, like we outlined earlier in this chapter. There are also other creative ways of finding out what you do and don't want to do (in our opinion, knowing what doesn't work is incredibly valuable). For example, seek out interesting volunteer opportunities, try to do some job shadowing, or seek mentoring from someone in a profession that appeals to you. If you have a more definite idea of something you'd like, try internships or co-op programs. The most important thing is to do your research. Don't be afraid to try new and different things, things you never thought about before lupus. Ask yourself and research some of the hard questions, like those in the following list: you may be surprised at your answers. **You are not your disease, but it is simply a part of your journey**. You can discover a career path that is right for you and that coincides instead of conflicting with your lupus path.

The other important aspect to keep in mind is that in order to maintain your health and your ability to work throughout your life, some creativity and flexibility is required. Always consider that you need to continuously balance your lupus life (after clarifying exactly what this means to you) as well as possible. Unfortunately, lupus is an unpredictable disease, and symptom management may sometimes interfere with your career, as will an unexpected flare-up. The key to career and lupus management is to have options so that you can adjust as required. Thus, you may need to reevaluate your career path at different times in your life. You may need to come up with creative solutions, such as working from home and/or developing new skills. Don't be discouraged by the challenges that lie ahead. Your task is to find out what works for you, for your career, and for your lupus.

You might have had a plan prior to being diagnosed with lupus, and we acknowledge that it is hard to deviate from that plan, and even harder to feel like you have to start all over again. However, changing career directions can be positive! Now you can establish new goals, such as really focusing on achieving work–life balance, working reasonable hours, choosing an appropriate career, and focusing on what you could do instead of what you should do. You are no longer limited by the expectations of others or those of your pre-lupus self. You can try new things and explore new options. You can now choose to do what interests you and fits into your life. Your life is not your job, nor is it your lupus. Your life is your own, and it contains a lot of different and interesting facets and parts. Lupus will certainly influence our goals and dreams, but we are the ones who ultimately choose the quality of our lives.

Some key career questions to ask yourself:
• What are you passionate about?
• What issues do you feel are really important?
• What do you do in your spare time that makes your life better?
• What topics would you like to learn more about?
• What are the skills that you possess?
• What skills would you like to improve?
• What are your best abilities?
• Where do you want to live?
• What are your financial goals?
• How does your family factor in?
• Do you want to/can you work part-time? Full-time?

- What are your ideal working hours?
- How much and what kind of training are you prepared to do in order to reach your career goal?
- Do you like working with people?
- Do you like working with numbers?
- How comfortable are you using technology?
- How do you feel about commuting? What are your commuting options?
- Do you want to work in an office or outdoors?
- Do you want to work from home?
- Are you more effective working independently or in a team-based environment? Or a combination of both?

Pursuing Your Career Path

The next things to consider, once you have chosen your career path and have completed the associated educational requirements, are choosing an appropriate employer and approaching them for employment.

When selecting an appropriate employer, there are some aspects pertaining to a company and/or a potential manager that are key to ensuring your success in your new position while maintaining your health. Specifically, it is helpful to identify companies that have done the following: taken proactive steps to recruit people with disabilities (such as federally regulated employers); made their diversity policies public; sponsored community initiatives; accommodated other individuals with disabilities; and have diversity equity officers on staff. This is not to say that you cannot look into jobs with other organizations. They would still be required to provide the necessary accommodations (or they may refuse you employment for what are possibly unjust reasons), however, best-practice employers would already have experience with putting accommodations into place, and therefore may be more willing to focus on your strengths throughout the hiring process.

Jodie has some insights into finding an appropriate employer that will likely surprise you, as they did her when she first discovered them. She attended a workshop run by the University of Toronto Career Centre on ways of finding employment. Those in attendance learned that **the most effective ways to find a job include: asking acquaintances for leads, walking into agencies, cold-calling/emailing organizations about possible job openings, and networking**. Conversely, the least effective ways to find a job include Internet job searching, random mailing, newspaper advertisements, and employment agencies. Employers tend to hire from – in order of priority – within their organization, or from proven applicants (typically connected with current employees), screened applicants (those for whom they already have a CV), and those who have responded to an advertisement. However, individuals looking for jobs tend to use the least effective ways to find a job (Internet job searching, responding to an advertisement, etc.). **Most individuals seeking employment use the simplest and least time-consuming method(s); meanwhile, employers are seeking employees who are prepared to invest in the most time-consuming method(s).**

Not surprisingly, networking is the number one way to find employment. We have all heard that it is not what you know, but *who you know*. Jodie has experienced this first-hand. The majority of her past and present jobs have been obtained through important personal and professional contacts, while the CVs she has dropped off randomly have gone unanswered. However, networking is more complex than most people would imagine. It is an ongoing process of developing and maintaining personal and professional relationships, and is mutually beneficial to both parties involved. Networking is not about asking for a job, but can provide leads that uncover job possibilities. It is just as important to maintain your current contacts as it is to develop and build your existing network, particularly as your career aspirations become clearer and/or change due to other life experiences. A key aspect of establishing and broadening your contacts is organization. Keep a list and/or database that records names, addresses, information about where you met them, and of course, what they do. Keep this list updated, because you just never know when you might need your contacts! One way to develop and maintain contacts is to use LinkedIn™.

Get Ready for the Job Hunt!

To get the most out of your job-hunting expedition, it's important to be organized about everything related to the job-search process. Make a 'Career Binder' so that you can keep and file everything from your résumés, CVs, contacts, career questionnaire results, and job advertisements, as well as a list of jobs you have applied to and followed up on. Keep a calendar to ensure that you are on schedule and that you will be applying for jobs at the right time, in addition to following-up with employers where you have applied. Job postings generally have deadlines, and it is often beneficial to follow up a couple of weeks later. Sometimes you will be informed of an upcoming posting, so leave a reminder for yourself in your calendar. Keep organized! **Trying to find a job is a job!** After all that, you can now add 'Being Organized" as a skill on your resume!

Once you have some ideas about what you want to do, and you are well organized, you now have to seek out the jobs you want. The most important step here is *research*. Make sure to know as much about the position and the organization as possible. Most organizations have websites that you can browse, but don't hesitate to speak to human resources (HR) personnel or to people inside the organization to determine what skills and attitudes are required of its employees. A great strategy to really research a company and job opportunities is to contact the HR department or someone in the organization and ask if you can have an informational interview. An informational interview tends to be an informal way for you to meet someone within the company, learn more about what the company does and what the company needs and what you can offer. This "insider" information can help you determine if this would be a suitable environment for you. Try not to rely solely on information that is presented in the job advertisement. Try your best to dig deeper, to see how you might fit in and how you can maximize your chances of being hired.

Hire me! How to maximize your résumé/ CV

Your résumé is essentially a very brief way of establishing a connection between yourself and a potential employer. As such, your résumé must be tailored to fit the demands of the job that you are seeking. That is why researching the organization and the position is so important. Your résumé should show that you "match" what is required of a potential employee. Be sure to highlight experiences and skills that are relevant to the work, such as language proficiency for tutoring or a Bronze Cross for lifeguarding. You may even have several résumé/CV formats to reflect different types of positions that interest you. Provide key examples of achievements and use strong verbs to illustrate your actions. Don't just say that you worked on a project. Be clear regarding your contribution. Did you coordinate, manage, or organize a part of or even the entire project?

One of the concerns about having a chronic illness is that you may feel that your experience may not measure up. Perhaps it took you a bit longer to finish your schooling, or perhaps there are gaps in your job timelines because you were dealing with major flare-ups. Don't get discouraged. Keep your résumé focused on the tasks you accomplished and the skills you developed. Be honest, and if your résumé seems a little bare, highlight skills that you developed during your time not being a student or being employed. You would be surprised how many management and self-advocacy skills you can develop through interactions with the health-care system! **This does not mean that you need to disclose your diagnosis, but simply means that there are resourceful ways of explaining gaps in your résumé.** So, think creatively, not only about your paid work, but also about your volunteer experiences and leisure activities. Career counselors can help you refine your résumé content and terminology, and they can also help you identify key skills and experiences.

There are several résumé templates and examples online, but the important thing is that your résumé should reflect *you*. Résumé writing is not easy and is a continual process involving regular updates and consultation. Be precise, concise, persuasive, professional, and most important of all: maintain a positive attitude! Job opportunities tend to appear when you least expect them, so always have an updated and edited personal "résumé skeleton" that can be filled in and sculpted to fit any potential job scenario.

Résumé or Curriculum Vitae (CV)?

A résumé applies for work in any area. It is usually a brief document (1–2 pages). A résumé includes an initial "Summary of Strengths" section and has subheadings such as Work Experience, Skills, Education, and more.

A CV generally aims at work in academic or research sectors. A CV is a longer document (it can be several pages, depending on your experience) and often includes extensive information on research publications, conference presentations, and fellowships.

E-résumés

Online résumés should include keywords that are being searched by the employer. Some keywords need to be in a separate section.
Résumés can be emailed as an attachment or included in the body of the email in plain text format. Find out what the employer's policy is on accepting attachments.

Hire me! Get ready for your interview

At some point in the job-hunting process you may be called in for an interview to further verify the information contained within your résumé, and to see how your personality and life philosophies might fit with your potential employer. Once again, the key skills needed for a successful interview are research and preparation. Be sure to learn as much as you can about the organization, and refer to this information during the interview. Potential employers are always impressed when you have taken the time to get to know them. The next step is to anticipate as many questions as possible that the employer may ask. Write down all the potential questions that you can think of, and practice your answers. The most common questions that employers include are behavioral-situational questions, wherein they will ask for a specific example of how you handled a situation in the past. Try to make your response sound like a story, using specific examples from your past to show how you used your skills and abilities to solve a problem. A good way to structure these responses is by using the SPARE template: **S**ituation or **P**roblem, **A**ction or behavior, **R**esult, and **E**nthusiasm. The situation or problem is the beginning of your story, where you outline what exactly the issue was (make sure that it fits the criteria of what the interviewer is asking). The majority of your story is the actions that you took and behaviors that you displayed to solve the issue. The result or outcome details how the issue was resolved. Be sure to conclude your story by enthusiastically stating how you really enjoyed the challenge. One interview preparation tactic involves thinking of potential questions that you may be asked, and then writing down your response using the SPARE template. In addition, **never underestimate the power of doing mock interviews with trusted and knowledgeable friends and family members.** They will be able to help you identify and address not only appropriate answers to likely questions, but also any nervous habits that you might have, such as twiddling your thumbs, fixing your hair, or not making eye contact. Employers are anxious to examine not only your verbal, but also your nonverbal skills during an interview.

Another key quality is confidence. Have pride in who you are and what you have accomplished. Dealing with a chronic illness is not easy, and as a result, you will have already developed a strong determination and personal resilience. Even though you may feel inadequate, because it is possible that managing your lupus has already taken a toll on your qualifications and experiences (and your self-esteem), now is the time to implement your creativity. All of your experiences (paid or unpaid, or even leisure!) can serve as examples of how you solved a problem, or developed your time management skills, or negotiated with another person. Never underestimate the skills learnt through navigating the health-care system! Adopt a flexible and innovative approach when appraising and marketing your own talents. Look at what you have already done with your life, and feel good about that; know that if you were successful before, you can certainly be successful again. During your interview, be positive and enthusiastic that you are embarking on this journey – your determination and bright outlook will only enhance the experience. For tips on telling your employer and your colleagues about your condition, or if your condition is visible and you are concerned about your interview, see the "You're Hired – Now What?" section that follows for advice on disclosure of information.

Sample Interview Questions and Answers

1. Potential Interview Question: Why has it taken you so long to finish your school program?

Sample Answer: Education is so costly that I decided to reduce my course load and take additional time to complete the requirements towards my degree, in order to have increased flexibility in my schedule for part-time employment without jeopardizing my course grades.

2. Potential Interview Question: Why has it taken you so long to find a job?

Sample Answer: I was really focused on trying to find the "right" job. I was really searching for an opportunity where my qualifications and personality would match the requirements of the job, and the goals of work projects. Over the past while, I have done a lot of research about this industry. I have gone to several informational interviews and I've even taken some courses to upgrade my skills. It was very beneficial to have this time to explore, and now I am prepared and ready for the right opportunity.

3. Potential Interview Question: Why did you leave your last job?

Sample Answer: To be honest, my last job wasn't the most effective fit at that time. I have done a lot of research about this industry, and about this company in particular. I have thoroughly reviewed the requirements for this position, and I can offer several examples showing that I have the necessary experience and skill sets to do this job effectively.

4. Potential Interview Question: What are your goals?

Sample Answer: Based on my personal qualifications and what I know about your company, I actually have both short- and long-term goals that I would like to accomplish. Right now, I would like to contribute to the project team, where I feel that my skills and personality will really be a benefit. My long-term goal will depend on how the company grows and develops, and I would like to grow and develop with this company.

5. Potential Interview Question: This job may periodically require long hours to meet deadlines. What flexibility do you have that will enable you to meet the requirements of your position?

Sample Answer: As you may have noticed from the experiences listed on my résumé, once I have dedicated myself to a particular endeavor, I am fully committed to seeing the project through to completion. If this requires working long hours once in a while, I will do what is necessary. What kind of compensation is provided during these circumstances? For example, am I able to bank the extra hours, or are there other similar benefits?

You're Hired – Now What?

Congratulations on choosing a career and finding a job. However, the challenges do not end here! All people who have recently been hired are placed under strict scrutiny during a probation period, which is already a highly stressful time given you are learning all the different roles in your new position. This stress can be heightened for individuals with a chronic health condition, sometimes as a result of worrying about whether your health will remain stable, and what to do should your employer find out about your condition. Therefore, it is also important to be familiar with the workplace rules regarding sick days and medical appointments, so that you know what to expect and what you can negotiate during the hiring process. Furthermore, it is really important to be aware of whether or not you have to disclose that you have lupus. Jodie's own struggles in trying to develop her disclosure policy led her to attend a very informative workshop at the University of Toronto's Career Centre regarding disclosure in the workplace for individuals with chronic health conditions. They provided feedback regarding different disclosure scenarios, as well as pros and cons associated with each scenario.

First, it is important to remember that in most countries (especially in Canada, thanks to the Canadian Human Rights legislation), people have the right to request accommodations in the workplace, as long as implementing those accommodations do not cause 'undue hardships' to the company, defined as being too expensive or too hard for the employer to put into place. Second, the process of deciding which accommodations you need requires some reflection and some investigation on your part. Identifying the need for accommodations is based upon personal resources, as well as the work environment. In relation to personal resources, you need to have a good understanding of your disability, your strengths and weaknesses, solutions that have worked in the past, and functional limits that might impede your ability to complete job tasks. **In relation to the work environment, you need to reflect on job demands, equipment you are expected to operate, limitations that might impede you from completing tasks and/or accessing your workplace,**

and how accommodations would improve your performance. Being able to identify how you can improve your situation, how your employer can improve your situation, and how these changes will improve your job performance is imperative to the likelihood of your new employer agreeing to meet all of your identified needs.

Answering these important questions about your personal resources and your work environment can help lead to your 'personal disclosure policy'. Although you have likely worked out how to discuss (or not discuss) your chronic condition with new acquaintances, explaining your condition to an employer is different. Other issues to consider when developing your personal disclosure policy include:

1. Are you required to take a placement test (for example, a language proficiency test) prior to being hired? If so, will you require special accommodations for testing?

If the answer is 'yes,' you will likely have to disclose your condition to those conducting the test. However, these tests are typically not hosted by the company you are approaching for employment. Therefore, your disclosure of your illness to those who are actually conducting the testing session (and getting the necessary accommodations to ensure your successful completion of the testing) should not affect the hiring process. If the company you are approaching for employment is administering the test, this is typically handled by their human resources department, who should use discretion when sharing this personal information with your potential direct supervisor throughout the hiring process.

2. Do you think your safety might be at stake if you do not disclose?

If your condition involves events such as seizures that require emergency medical intervention, it might be best to disclose to at least one individual who will be working in close proximity. To be really discrete, while still ensuring your safety, you may even just tell a few trusted colleagues that you wear a MedicAlert™ bracelet/necklace (or watch/sport band) and that should something happen, you would appreciate their notifying the emergency personnel when they arrive.

3. How visible is your condition?

If you use any physical aids, such as a wheelchair, and are asked questions about your condition, you might be more prone to disclosing about your condition. However, you are never required to disclose precisely what your condition is, even if there are obvious physical signs that you have additional health needs. You are only required to answer questions about how your condition may (or may not) affect your job productivity, and what accommodations you need to ensure that you are able to fulfill your roles and responsibilities.

4. Will your condition possibly affect the interview and/or hiring process?

This is very similar to the previous item. If you feel that using an aid like a walker will affect your chances of being hired, or your ability to participate in the interview process (for example if it's a group interview or involves skill-testing), or that the interviewer will be uncomfortable with a visible marker (such as a speech impediment or a facial rash), it may be best to acknowledge your condition, and then to quickly divert the conversation to your strengths, your achievements, and how you exceed the expectations outlined in the job description.

5. Can your needs be met without disclosing?

If your needs can be met without disclosing, for example, flexible work hours, then there is no need to disclose. If, however, the accommodations you require are likely to raise questions about why they are needed, then disclosing that you have a chronic health condition might be necessary. However, even then, you are never required to name your condition, or to explain how it affects your life.

If your employer sees your strengths, and sees how you have been able to manage meeting other goals in your life (through having the same accommodations you are currently requesting), they are more likely to perceive you in a positive light. Even if it is obvious that you have a medical condition (for example, you use a wheelchair), your employer legally cannot ask direct questions about it. Of course, after you have worked for a few months, have passed your probation period, have proven that you can meet job expectations, and have developed a positive relationship with your employer, you may decide to disclose, having built a mutually trusting relationship. If you are facing some challenges at work and experiencing difficulty with certain tasks, you may feel that communicating with your boss or co-workers might be beneficial. People are usually reasonable if you explain that you have a medical condition that might make some duties difficult at times. It is possible that your workload or timelines can be adjusted so that everyone can accomplish the task in an appropriate manner. However, whether to discuss your medical condition with your bosses and or co-workers, and in what detail, is ultimately up to you.

If your supervisor is not reasonable when you tell him/her about your need for accommodations, you have a couple of options: (1) tell someone who is higher up than your supervisor, such as the general manager, or a union representative; (2) file a complaint with a human rights advocacy group/council (e.g., the Canadian Human Rights Commission) if you want to pursue legal action that would basically force your supervisor to provide the accommodations you require; or (3) find another job with an employer who is more understanding and accepting of different people's needs.

From our personal experiences, the experiences of other young people with chronic health conditions, and recommendations from employers and career counselors, we can confirm that there are two primary disclosure scenarios. The first includes discussing accommodations after you have been accepted for the position and are in the midst of negotiating your work contract. First, if you know you will need special accommodations to meet your job expectations, and these accommodations will require disclosure of a chronic health condition, it is ideal to disclose upon signing your contract. The benefits of this scenario are: (1) demonstrating that you are legally aware that you are not required to disclose, until necessary, thereby informing your employer that you are aware of your legal and human rights; (2) your employer will not be able to change any previously discussed terms of your contract, because you are now in the driver's seat in terms of negotiations; (3) you can be certain that your employer has hired you based on merit, not merely to meet their quota for hiring a certain number of individuals with special needs; and (4) your employer will notice that you have put some thought into how to disclose your situation, and which accommodations are needed (and why). Your new employer will translate these skills into the "attention to detail" that you will likely use on different tasks you will be taking on in your new job. Therefore, you will need to be prepared to explain exactly which accommodations are needed, why you need them, and how they will ensure that you can meet your job expectations.

The second scenario entails waiting until you require a special accommodation before you disclose. This scenario is most commonly utilized by individuals who are diagnosed with a cyclical condition, such as lupus, which is characterized by periods of stability interspersed with bouts of illness. Most likely, when you are applying for a job, you are in a period of relative stability, and therefore you may not require any accommodations. However, given the unpredictable nature of lupus, you will likely experience a flare-up at some point during the course of your employment. By disclosing only when accommodations become necessary: (1) you are exercising your human rights; (2) you will have already demonstrated your dedication to your position; (3) you will likely have a clear idea of which accommodations are necessary based on past job performance; and (4) you have quite possibly spent enough time in your position to qualify for special disability-related and sick-leave benefits offered by both your employer and the government.

As previously mentioned, in any situation of disclosure, you are ultimately in control of deciding whether to disclose, and how much information to share. We encourage everyone to take the time to reflect on the different questions and scenarios presented in this section, and to start to develop their own 'personal disclosure policy.' Once you are in the market for full-time employment, it will be a lot less stressful to have already decided upon your personal preference – searching for a job is stressful enough!

Summer and Part-time Employment

Most young adults will have the opportunity to gain their own income, whether working part-time throughout the school year, or full-time during the summer months. However, there are some questions to consider if you are challenged by a chronic health condition. Specifically, if you are a student, will you be able to manage your school expectations and household responsibilities, maintain your health, and keep some time free for your friends if you take on a part-time job? You might need to review how you have been managing everything else in your life before adding another stressor. If you are in high school and have always maintained decent grades, enjoyed good friendships, and haven't experienced too much stress at home with your parents, then you might consider adding a part-time job to your routine. If you have just begun post-secondary education, even if you were able to manage your health, school, and part-time or summer vacation work as a high school student, you may need to give serious consideration to completing at least your first semester prior to seeking part-time employment. University and college expectations are much higher compared to those during high school, even before considering the additional stress of possibly living on your own for the first time, being in a new city, making new friends, seeing a new doctor, and everything else that goes with starting a new chapter in your life. Although these are all positive changes, any change is stressful, and we need time for our bodies and minds to adjust to the new circumstances.

Even during the summer months, some of us will not be able to manage being employed full-time, or even part-time, while maintaining our health. This may be due to either the challenges of working while struggling with an illness, or needing the time to refuel after a busy school year. We need to acknowledge that although we are just like other people in many ways, we each have special needs, and must respect our limits, otherwise there could be some severe consequences – possibly long term.

Even if you are no longer a student, these same considerations apply. Some of us will not be able to manage full-time employment, and will therefore only seek part-time employment, even following graduation. Our employment status might change once we find that we are able to manage part-time employment. However, this will likely fluctuate along with our health – something we are all too familiar with. This is all part of having a flexible, long-term career plan, and being willing to explore different job options within our chosen career path and field of interest.

Some important considerations for everyone seeking summer and/or part-time employment relate to disclosure and requesting special accommodations (including seeking employment out of the hot sun). Through personal experience, Jodie has learned that the majority of employers are not as concerned about hiring students with chronic health conditions for part-time or summer employment compared with full-time positions. That said, most employers will also say that it is best to only disclose if you have to. As mentioned earlier in the section "You're Hired – Now What?," there are many reasons why someone might choose to disclose at different stages of the hiring process, but we all need to remember that disclosure is never mandatory (in Canada). Likewise, the same approaches to finding employment that were mentioned in the section "Pursuing your Career Path" are relevant to finding summer and part-time jobs – including using your connections.

A final thought about part-time and summer employment: although we all enjoy the monetary advantages of working, there are also other benefits. Whether paid or voluntary, part-time and summer jobs offer the opportunity to try out possible career paths, to make connections towards future jobs, and to develop skills that may not be taught in the classroom. They offer the opportunity to interact socially with others, to improve your physical and psychological well-being, and to "get out and about" and meet new people. When considering job options, reflect upon the different benefits from potential positions. For example, one summer Jodie decided to take a $4/hour pay cut from the previous year to be able to work in her chosen field of counseling. This later benefited her by being an important component to Jodie's graduate school application, and the skills that she learnt that summer are some that she still uses, even after having completed her master's degree.

So, when addressing your career options, always keep your health in mind, but never give up on your goals! Even with lupus, you can still have a fabulous career and life!

Useful Sources of Information

Canadian Human Rights Commission:
Administers the **Canadian Human Rights Act** and is responsible for ensuring compliance with the **Employment Equity Act**. Both laws ensure that the principles of equal opportunity and non-discrimination are followed in all areas of federal jurisdiction.
www.chrc-ccdp.ca/default-en.asp

High School/University/College Career Centers:
Offer services for building résumés, practicing interviews, career-personality matching questionnaires, and sessions with career counselors to discuss options, given the unique challenges for each individual.

Lupus Canada:
Meet others who have lived through similar challenges to discuss options, frustrations, and shared experiences.
www.lupuscanada.org

NEADS (National Educational Association of Disabled Students)
They offer job-strategy forums for students with disabilities.
www.neads.ca

Disability Related Policy in Canada:
To help people with disabilities to understand how government policy,
especially at the federal level, makes decisions that shape their lives.
www.disabilitypolicy.ca/index_english.php

Disability Vocational Rehabilitation Program:
The Canada Pension Plan Disability Vocational Rehabilitation Program is
designed to help people who receive a Canada Pension Plan disability benefit
to return to work.
www.hrsdc.gc.ca/eng/isp/pub/factsheets/vocrehab.shtml

Enable Link:
Linking people with disabilities with a world of resources
www.enablelink.org

Career Joy:
Find the right career for you.
www.careerjoy.com

Career Options:
A student resource that includes vital career search tips from experts, industry
profiles, a career search section, co-op and internship information, and more.
For both secondary and post-secondary students across Canada.
www.careeroptionsmagazine.com

MONEY & FINANCES

Stash Your Cash

Many people do not like dealing with money, but in our opinion you have to be comfortable tackling your finances. A person with lupus must be especially careful with their financial planning, because this illness can become unexpectedly severe, and may interfere with your ability to work and earn an income. Jessica has found that saving some money is the most important financial strategy to use, just in case she is not able to work at some point. Saving some money is recommended for everyone, but many people don't save anything at all! **If you have lupus, you cannot afford to not save**. Planning ahead is critical when you have lupus, because you will not be able to rely on ongoing good health and a continuous cash flow like most other people. In fact, no one should rely on the expectation of perfect health, because those of us with lupus know that you can get bad news regarding your health at any time in your life. That is why you must try to plan as best as you can. Financial planning may seem like a tiring task, but it does not have to be that hard. Keep in mind that dealing with a flare-up is extremely hard, and you've already been through that! The good news is that if you are careful and realistic with your money you will likely end up in much better financial health than your so-called healthy peers. In Jessica's experience, having good financial management skills helps keep her lupus under control because she is not constantly worrying about money. She is able to manage her stress because she manages her money. This feeling is priceless.

Saving is the cornerstone of a sound financial future. You must continuously save something, *anything*, in order to guarantee that you can afford the things you need. In order to save, you must live below your means. Living below your means equals living your life and still having some extra money without using credit (cards or loans). One effective strategy you can try is to 'pay yourself first'. Each time you get paid, the amount of money that you have decided to save should go straight into a special account, so that you won't spend it. This is far better than waiting to see what's left over at the end of the month. The money that you have "paid yourself" can then go toward short-term savings (emergency fund), longer-term savings (future fund), and bigger-ticket items. How much money should go into each of these categories depends on many different factors such as your age, lifestyle, income, goals, etc. These are personal decisions that you can make with the help of trusted individuals, like your financial advisor or family, but always remember that when it comes to your money, the final decisions are up to you!

To know how much money you have to put into savings when paying yourself first, you can start by tracking (using a spreadsheet or online tool) everything you spend over, say, a three-month period, right down to a dollar on a pack of gum! You should also track how much money you have coming in each month. Make sure you have enough to pay for your essential items (rent, food, medication), and then put the rest of your money into different "pots" for savings. Once you know how much money you can place into these different "pots", you can set up automatic transfers to pay these amounts into your different savings accounts each month When you are young, you are so focused on aspects of your current life such as school, friends, work, and relationships that it is incredibly easy to not think about what seems like the very distant future. When you are a young person with lupus, you are even less likely to be thinking about the future because you are too busy focusing on just getting through each day, and possibly dealing with a severe flare-up. We both agree that dealing with your illness in the here and now is a key priority, but the future is closer than you think. So, while it is hard to imagine your future while you are struggling in the present, that future will inevitably arrive. For those with lupus, you cannot ignore the fact that your illness may become so severe that you may not be able to continue to earn money for long periods, and you will need to cover your expenses. So, while you are healthy and earning an income, please do your best to put some money away each month, even if it is just a little bit. It will add up over time.

In addition to saving for emergencies, try to start saving for your future goals, whatever they may be. If your goal is post-secondary education, then go for it! Check out the School & Education chapter for ideas and tips. No matter what your future goals are, don't let lupus stop you! **You can achieve (and finance) any dream that you have.** You can set a series of savings goals, and celebrate when you reach each milestone. It will likely make you feel so much better and secure knowing that you have a plan in place. Do not underestimate the power of this kind of security. That feeling is worth every cent in your emergency fund.

The good news for those with lupus is that due to modern medicine and careful management, you will likely live to a ripe old age. The bad news is, you will need to be able to meet all your expenses in your old age. In order to save for the future, you have to start saving as soon as you begin to receive an income. Where and how you choose to "store" your money is your choice. There are many future savings options available, some of which can vary depending on where you live. There are options that will give you guaranteed returns, whereby you will get back the money you put in, plus some interest. There are also stocks and mutual funds (collection of stocks), which carry more risk, because it's possible to lose some of your money, but they also offer the possibility of bigger returns over time. For those living in Canada, the Canadian government offer options whereby you can register your investments in a Registered Retirement Savings Plan (RRSP), or Tax Free Savings Account. Go to www.cra.gc.ca for more details, or visit your local financial institution.

This is a personal decision that only you can make, because it has to be the right decision for you, your current status, your daily needs, and your future goals. Be sure to do your research and/or talk to financial experts that you trust. Don't let anyone bully you into doing something you don't want to do or feel uncomfortable doing. Assess yourself honestly, and decide what your priorities are. Then, do your research, and choose the best option for you and your money. Just like lupus, finances depend on the individual, and may be difficult to predict. Keep monitoring the growth of your long-term savings, knowing that you will always have the option to tweak them if it becomes necessary, and as you see fit.

Based on Jessica's experience, saving for what is to come is a fabulous strategy, because financing her future not only reduces her current daily stresses, but she does not fret about her life 50 years from now. With sound financial planning, both the present and the future seem bright!

Buyer Beware

Of course, everyone needs to spend some money in order to live, and for this spending, **it is a good idea to prioritize, plan, and save for everything that you purchase**. For example, if you want a new pair of jeans, a dryer, and a vacation, you need to determine the order of priority, and then figure out the best way to set aside some money for these things. This may seem pointless, given that we live in a consumer-driven world of instant gratification, credit cards, and payday loans. However, if you don't want to be saddled with never-ending repayments at crushing interest rates (which will surely cause stress), you need to save up the money for each item you want, and only buy what you can afford with the money you have saved. While this may seem really difficult, it can be done. Jodie managed to save some money while studying and living on a student loan – and it is well known that student loans are below the poverty line! (The amount given to students through government student loans is typically less than what has been calculated by the government as being necessary for an individual to buy what is needed to live – such as shelter and food.) Always remember that easy access to credit (i.e. money that is not your own) is a relatively recent phenomenon, and that your parents and grandparents existed fairly well without credit. If you need to purchase something using a loan (like a car, which is both a large purchase and often a necessity for employment), then please take the time to do some research and get the best possible deal. In addition, make sure you stand your ground and negotiate for the lowest interest rate that you can obtain. The most important thing is to have a plan whenever you go shopping. This will help you stay on track, and only purchase the items that you truly need and can afford.

In order to purchase items that you will need in the future, you may have to consider sacrificing a few items now. When considering the purchase of non-essential items, make sure you are buying these items for the right reasons. Do you want to buy something because you are bored, stressed, or sad? Are you worried, anxious, or depressed due to your illness, or perhaps for some other reason? Or do you want to buy this item because you really need it, or you really love it, or it will really bring you happiness? Although it is certainly fun to blow all your money and live for today, especially when you have a painful and unpredictable illness like lupus, repeating these actions over and over again will only hurt you in the future. Jessica loves to shop, and admits that it is a soothing experience. She also knows how hard it is to refrain from buying all the things that her friends are buying. However, we all know that there is no purchase that will cure lupus, or loneliness, or whatever else it is that you are suffering from. Having some money saved up will not get rid of lupus either, but it may reduce some of your anxieties. That said, living a balanced life is key. So spend your money wisely on the things that are most important to you and that bring you joy. Say no to the stuff that will just weigh you down with debt and stress. Peace of mind is worth more than any number of new pairs of shoes.

Balanced Budget = Balanced Life

There are very few people in the world who truly love to budget their cash flow and stick to their spending plan. The rest of us just have to suck it up and do it. We can guess what you're thinking right now: "Having lupus is bad enough, so why do I have to budget too?" We agree that budgeting may seem boring, but you need to have a plan if you have an illness, because at some point you will incur certain expenditures that will be crucial to your quality of life. For example, most people have a budget with the following categories: housing, transportation, life (food, personal items, clothing), debt repayment, other, etc., but if you have lupus, you also need to factor medical expenses into your budget. Jodie offers some great suggestions in the Tips to Reduce Medical

Expenses section later in this chapter on how to save money on the things that you need if you have lupus, but you still need to include this in your budget. Medications (both prescription and nonprescription), transportation costs to visit doctors, massage appointments, new clothes if your weight has been fluctuating, sunscreen, etc., are just a few of the items that you may need to allow for, because they can add up over time.

Budgeting may seem restrictive and boring, but it can actually provide you with a lot of freedom. When you know how much money is going where, you are free to really enjoy spending the money that is earmarked for the things you love. Thanks to modern technology (such as apps and spreadsheets), creating and maintaining a budget is really easy. The best way to create your own budget (or one for your household) is to keep track all of your spending for a few months, recording absolutely everything that you purchase, and how much it costs. Then, you need to develop a plan (using the categories that apply to you) to make sure that your income is at least equal to the amount you are spending. It seems simple enough, but it can be hard to stay on budget (trust us!). Still, it's well worth the effort, because the rewards of a balanced budget include a good night's sleep, less stress and anxiety, and feeling more in control of your life. Balancing your budget is a key component of successful money management, and this can only help you to better manage your lupus.

Benefits@Work

Working has many great benefits, which we have already explored in the Careers & Employment chapter, but two areas that we did not talk about so much are the financial and medical aspects. Specifically, once you reach a point in your life when you are working full-time, you will likely have access to medical benefits, which is a huge relief to those of us with chronic medical conditions. However, it is still important to review the package that is provided by your employer to ensure that all of your needs are being met. Sometimes this information is available through your human resources department, but at other times you may need to call the insurance company directly for a complete review. If the medical insurance package that you are paying for out of your weekly paycheck is not meeting all of your needs, discuss your options with your supervisor, the HR department, and the insurance company to see if you can boost the existing package to include items that will cover your specific concerns.

Likewise, it is important to review the percentage of your paycheck that is going towards taxes, your pension, and other such items. Although there is typically a set percentage, this is usually flexible at the request of the employee, so be sure to get all the facts about where your money is going, and ask for any changes that might help meet your commitments at various stages of your life and your future goals. For example, you may choose to alter your contribution amount to your pension plan when your situation changes (i.e. getting married, having kids, etc.). The point is to be proactive and to ask questions. **You earned this money, and you have the right to know where it is going**.

The other really important area related to work is when, for health-related reasons, you are unable to work. There are a couple of different scenarios regarding this situation. First, if you have been working for a reasonable amount of time, your employer might be able to provide a short-term disability package. To become eligible, a doctor's note outlining the reason why you are unable to work for a set period and the expected date of your return to work will be required, and there may also be a special form for your doctor to complete. You are usually still able to access the other health benefits offered through your employer's insurance program while taking this time off. If your employer does not offer short-term disability (or sickness benefits), there are disability support options that are provided through the national and provincial government. However, the additional health benefits offered through these government assistance programs vary quite a bit. Most of these government programs are accessible through online applications and/or through an in-person application at offices in all major cities. Be sure to do your own research and review all the available benefits to ensure that you access the most suitable options for your particular needs (for example, www.canadabenefits.gc.ca for Canadians).

We understand that there is a possibility that your condition will not permit you to work full-time for your entire working life. If this is the case, it may be best to purchase disability insurance. If you are Canadian, you can apply for the Disability Support Program through your provincial government. This program offers medical coverage in addition to a minimal monthly income, but it takes the income of your partner (if you have one) into consideration, so not everyone is automatically eligible. There are lots of rules and conditions, so once again you will have to do your own research to see what is available and what would best meet your needs.

The bottom line is not to be afraid to ask questions about the support you have through your job, and to explore various forms of support available through your provincial/state and federal governments. If you don't ask, you won't know what you have access to – **advocate for yourself!** There is always an option that will ensure that your basic financial and medical needs are met.

Benefits@School

While you are attending school, there are fewer options regarding medical insurance and financial savings, mostly because you are in the process of studying (as opposed to working a paid job). When it comes to financing your studies, there is the option of borrowing money from the government or from a bank. There is also the option of scholarships and bursaries. Of course, the best option is to pay your way through your studies by working, if, and only if, your health permits it. For more information, see the School & Education chapter.

When it comes to medical insurance, students typically fall into one of two categories: (1) students are covered by their parents' medical insurance plan until the age of 25 (the exact age may vary depending on where you live and the type of plan) while studying full-time; or (2) students benefit from the medical insurance plan organized by their college or university for students who either do not have adequate coverage through their parents or are over the age of 25 or 26 years. In addition, some students who have medical benefits through either of the two options mentioned above choose to boost their coverage by subscribing to a provincial plan.

Tips to Reduce Medical Expenses

There are lots of ways to save money on your medical expenses. Some only involve a couple of dollars, but if you implement as many of the tips as possible (depending upon your own personal circumstances), those dollars can quickly add up! When it comes to the expensive medication that might be prescribed to manage your lupus, there are a couple of things to keep in mind.

1. Check with your rheumatologist, and with your other doctors, to see if they can provide any free samples.

2. Check with the drug manufacturer to see if they can either provide free samples or reduce the cost, based upon your personal financial situation.

3. Some pharmacies charge more than others for filling your prescription, so shop around to see who offers the best price. If your budget permits, try purchasing more than one month's worth of meds at a time. This will save you from paying the filling fee for each prescription every month. Some pharmacies charge $10 per prescription, so if you are taking 10 different medications, that's $100 per month in filling fees! If you can purchase a two-month supply each time, that's a potential annual saving of $600.

4. Some prescriptions are only covered by your health insurance if you are using the generic brand, so always ask your doctor for the generic version of any new medication.

NOTE: Sometimes the generic brand does not work, and you must use a name brand. If this is the case, have your doctor write a letter explaining why the generic brand did not work for your symptoms, and submit the letter to your medical insurance company. This could help get the medication covered for you.

5. Some prescriptions are expensive and are not covered by your medical insurance, but there are a couple of things you can try in this situation. First, your doctor can complete a Medical Exemption form. This can typically result in an insurance company providing at least some coverage. Second, if you only need to take a medication for a little while, then your doctor can write the prescription to reflect your limited use of that particular medication. Again, this can result in an insurance company agreeing to cover the cost of your medication.

6. A lot of people who take prescription medications also have to take vitamins and minerals to offset their body's failure to absorb nutrients properly. It can sometimes be cheaper to purchase these over-the-counter items with a prescription, so check with your insurance plan and with your pharmacy.

There are a couple of other things to keep in mind to help offset the cost of medication that is not covered by your health insurance, which often only covers 80% of costs.

First, some cities, like Ottawa, Canada, have additional support available through the city. These programs are intended for people who have no means of paying for extra medical expenses. There are qualification criteria, but if you qualify it can really help reduce your expenses.

Second don't forget to claim the cost of your medications on your taxes (at press time, in Canada you can claim 20%)! This is a great way of recouping at least some of the money you have had to pay throughout the year.

While we're on the subject of taxes, don't forget to keep all your receipts for medical expenses you have incurred throughout the year. You never know what you might be able to claim on your taxes. Some simple examples include expenses incurred in relation to travel to and from doctors' appointments, including meals and accommodation (the amount will vary depending on how far you have to travel and how long your appointment takes), and any equipment that your medical team recommends.

One more piece of advice: speak with the social worker attached to your medical clinic to find out more about what is available in your area. Part of the social worker's role within the hospital is to help ensure that individuals are able to pay for their medical needs, to help address work or school stressors, to ensure that you have adequate support at home, and to provide emotional support to you and your family. Social workers know that **there is always a solution, even if it means putting the patient in contact with several financial support options** to ensure that all of their medical requirements are accessible.

Financial Planners?

Your financial needs will invariably change throughout your life, and at some point, you may decide that you want specific and professional advice. Just like with medical advice, make sure that the person providing you with information is knowledgeable, credible, and trustworthy. Jessica has had several experiences with different financial advisors during various phases of her life. The variety of situations that she has experienced have ranged from not having lupus to having lupus, from being a student to being employed, and from being single to getting married. Selecting a financial advisor may seem trivial, but your financial health is very important to your overall health, so if you decide that you would like some professional financial advice, just like with health advice, be careful who you listen to, and trust your instincts. To health and prosperity!

Here are few 'Dos' and 'Don'ts' that we want to share with you based on our experiences:

Don't always go with the person who is provided for you. Some banks or institutions simply assign an advisor to you, but feel free to shop around. The right match is out there somewhere!

Don't be ashamed if you don't know all of the financial lingo. Speak up, ask questions, and make sure your advisor explains everything clearly and to your satisfaction.

Don't let anyone take advantage of you or your lupus. You are the client, and if your planner is pressuring you, you can leave them at any time.

Don't be afraid to ask as many questions as you want or need. Remember that you are the client, and you need to know what is going on with your money.

Don't schedule appointments with your advisor when you are experiencing a flare-up. You will make more informed decisions when you are feeling better.

Don't give up on your dreams just because you have lupus and your financial situation might not always be perfect. A good financial planner can help you to live the life you want and still do all the things that are most important to you.

Do make your own choices. It is your money, and you call the shots, so *you* are the one who must choose the person who will be advising you about your money.

Do explain your current situation clearly. Although you have to plan for the future, you also have to plan for the present, which includes such things as education, traveling, and possibly having a family.

Do be careful. If a so-called investment seems too good to be true, then it probably is.

Do your own research too! There are lots of good resources out there, and increasing your financial knowledge will only help you in the long run.

Do choose someone who you feel comfortable with. You should be able to feel that you trust this person, that you are able to discuss your financial situation openly with them, and that you can ask as many questions as you need.

Do be honest and realistic about your goals. Your planner will ask you a lot of questions about what you want to accomplish in the future. Try and have some ideas as a starting point, but you will likely discover a few things about yourself that you never considered as you map out your financial future with your planner!

STAYING ACTIVE

Lupus and an Active Lifestyle

Warning: not being active is a hazard to your health!

Every day, we are bombarded with the same message: exercise is good for us and being inactive is bad. You hear this on the news, you hear it from your friends and family, and you hear it from your doctor. It's like a broken record: Exercise! Exercise! Exercise! When all you want to do is take a nap! If you are like us, you are sick and tired of hearing that exercise will make you less sick and tired! However, while it is tempting to ignore those never-ending messages urging you to be more active, **if you have lupus, not exercising is not an option**. Although regular exercise is important for everyone, physical activity is a must if you have lupus. Not only does physical activity help reduce the negative impact of lupus, it is the key to achieving a healthier life overall. Furthermore, physical activity has the power to give us back our strength, endurance, and confidence that lupus can often take away.

Even a moderate amount of daily movement is exercise, and therefore a weapon in the fight against the effects of lupus. Exercise will invigorate your body and give you a sense of vitality and accomplishment. For patients with chronic back pain, instead of bed rest, daily moderate physical activity is now recommended to strengthen and stretch the back and shoulder muscles. The same advice applies to those patients with chronic fatigue syndrome – regular physical activity is recommended to help set a regular sleeping pattern by triggering the production of sleep-inducing hormones. For those of us with lupus, regular physical activity is recommended not only for the reasons already mentioned, but also to help with the body's absorption and circulation of medications, and to help combat some nasty side effects from those medications such as water retention and decreased bone density. Celebrate your body by moving it! Exercise not only provides physical benefits, but also provides several mental and emotional benefits that can help you cope with your illness. Here are just ten of the ways in which exercise can specifically benefit *you*!

1. **Helps maintain a healthy weight:** Regularly moving your body will help achieve and maintain a healthy weight. Achieving a healthy weight will reduce the stress on your joints, which is important, because as we all know, joint pain is a common and harmful aspect of lupus. Furthermore, many of us have to take corticosteroid drugs (such as prednisone), and two of the most common side effects of these medications are weight gain and reduced bone/muscle density. Because drastic weight gain is not generally good for our health, we really need to combat excess weight with exercise.

2. **Increases self-confidence and self-esteem:** Exerting yourself physically will make you feel really good, because you have just accomplished something. Accomplishing goals on a regular basis will make you feel stronger, and give you the sense that you can conquer anything that comes your way, such as that next lupus flare-up. Lupus has a dramatic impact on your self-esteem and self-confidence, and when you are diagnosed everyone keeps telling you what you can't do. Exercise (no matter how little) can give you back some of your power, because you are actually doing something!

3. **Promotes better sleep:** Exercise makes you more tired, and this can help you get a better night's sleep. Sleep is extremely important for preventing lupus flare-ups. Exercising can also help your body develop a regular sleeping pattern; just be careful not to exercise too close to bedtime, or you may have difficulty falling asleep. When we exercise regularly, our bodies want and need regular sleep to help them recover and reenergize.

4. **Strengthens our immune system:** Because many of us have to take drugs to suppress our overactive immune systems, it is important to do everything

we can to boost our immune systems. Having decent immune systems can help ward off minor illnesses (such as colds or infections) and prevent these "small" illnesses from progressing into full-blown sicknesses. Regular exercise helps our bodies to stay strong against germs.

5. **Gives you more energy:** Though exercise is tiring, it actually gives you more energy overall because your heart, lungs, and muscles become stronger over time. You feel energized after a workout because of the increased oxygen flowing throughout your body, and the changes in "feel-good" hormones. Moreover, your energy levels will likely be higher throughout the day. Not having enough energy to do basic things (as well as the things you love) is a major problem with lupus. Sometimes, just dealing with the lupus can drain you of your energy, but exercise can often restore that energy. While this may seem counterintuitive (expending energy in order to create more energy) doing regular exercise will definitely leave you feeling more alive.

6. **Builds strength:** It is very important that we maintain our strength in order to deal with lupus. Being physically strong will help support your joints and bones through the difficult times of lupus flare-ups. You also need to combat the reduction in your bone and muscle strength that is one of the common side effects of medication. Being stronger physically will make you feel stronger mentally and help you cope with this illness. Never underestimate the power that your enhanced physical capabilities can have in improving your self-esteem and optimism.

7. **Increases flexibility:** It is really important that our joints stay both strong and flexible. Flexibility can reduce joint pain, which is a common problem for those with lupus, in addition to preventing injuries.

8. **Reduces stress:** Most people feel really good after doing some form of

physical activity. When you exert yourself physically, you can eliminate a lot of stress and tension. Exercise can help you to relax, because while you are engaged in an activity, you are focusing on something other than your illness (and all the stress it creates in your life). Exercising also releases "feel-good" hormones, which helps reduce stress, anxiety, and depression, all of which are common in individuals with lupus.

9. **Keeps your heart strong:** We all need a strong heart so that it can keep pumping blood to the rest of our organs (lungs, brain, etc.). When one has lupus, having an efficiently functioning heart is essential in order to keep the rest of our bodies working effectively. Because many of the medications that we take can sometimes negatively impact our heart and our blood flow, we need to counteract these effects with exercise. If we want to have a healthy body and life, we have to have a healthy heart.

10. **Reduces the risk additional illness:** Exercise can help to prevent almost all forms of illness. Having lupus is hard enough (and most of us have lupus together with some other autoimmune illness), so it is important to do our best to stop our chances of developing any other chronic conditions.

Health in a Heartbeat

What is cardio and why is it important?

Cardiovascular activity (hereafter referred to as 'cardio') is any exercise that involves the heart and respiratory system. Cardio can do a lot of good things for your body, including lowering blood pressure, and reducing stress. It can help you burn calories (which can lead to losing weight), increase your resting metabolic level (which basically means the number of calories you burn while resting), and lower your risk for heart disease. Some other benefits of cardio were covered in the previous section.

While you have to make sure you do enough exercise to obtain these benefits, too much of a good thing can be harmful, so make sure you don't overdo it and put yourself at risk. Current recommendations are 30 minutes of exercise at least 5 days per week. The best way to make sure you are sticking to your limits is to pay attention to your body – are you totally out of breath, or in even worse pain than usual? Then ease off a bit and see what happens. Always pay attention to your body and how you are feeling. Remember that exercise is supposed to make you feel great!

Suggestions for cardio activities

There are countless cardio exercises that you can do, but before starting any exercise program, you should check with your doctor to make sure that you're good to go. Later, you can always consult a physiotherapist, dietician, or personal trainer at any time for advice on ways to reduce pain, increase activity, or increase benefits – safely.

Once you've been given the all clear by your doctor, it's important to do a warm-up followed by a light stretch prior to undertaking any activity. Warming up gradually increases your heart rate and gets your muscles moving, which greatly reduces your chances of injuring yourself. The best type of warm-up is to do the same exercise you will be doing, but more slowly, with less intensity, and/ or with lower weights if they're part of your routine.

As for specific cardio activities, there are plenty to choose from, the possibilities being virtually unlimited, but here are a few ideas to get you started. **The easiest and most accessible activity is walking** – for those of us with pain, it is easy on your joints, and for those of us who are unable to afford a gym membership, it is cheap. It can be done indoors or outdoors, and can easily be made more challenging by (1) moving more quickly, (2) increasing the range of motion of your legs, or (3) carrying weights. Of course, walking can easily progress to either hiking or running, or both. Hiking, or "walking on uneven terrain" as it is officially termed, presents your body with much more of a challenge than simply walking on city sidewalks or flat walking tracks, because your muscles have to work harder just to keep you balanced. In addition, walking in the forest increases the pleasure of being outdoors, compared with being surrounded by buildings and/or traffic. Research has shown that exercising with Mother Nature decreases depression, increases optimism, decreases anxiety, and improves circulation, along with many other positive side effects[2].

A few years ago, Jodie sustained a knee injury and was forced to hang up her gym shoes and take up walking, and soon came to enjoy her 30–60 minute daily walks around her neighborhood in Montreal. She discovered a lot that she didn't know existed, while taking in plenty of fresh air (well, as much as is possible in a large city). She couldn't wait for her daily excursion, particularly on those days when she was dragging her body around due to fatigue, or when her hips or knees had sharp pains, or when her head was foggy with stress. After a brisk walk, she was always left clear-headed, ready to tackle some more schoolwork, and her joints always felt better. So, pick up a pair of comfortable shoes and explore a new part of your home town/city today!

Some additional outdoor cardio exercise ideas include: dancing, bicycling, jumping rope, swimming, and skiing. Meanwhile, exercises to do indoors include treadmills, stationary bicycles, stair-climbers, rowing machines, elliptical trainers, ladder climbers, and yoga, as well as a large assortment of exercise classes.

Never underestimate what your body can do. Every exercise can be modified for all body types and abilities – take dancing, for example. Whether it's ballroom, classical ballet, modern tap, hip-hop, a religious celebration, or just a good night on the town with some friends, dancing is an excellent, universal form of exercise. Although Jodie has always loved to dance, she wasn't sure whether dancing could be for everyone, but after working with the Active Living Alliance for Canadians with Disabilities (ALACD), she learned that absolutely everyone can dance. ALACD offers unique programs to encourage young people of all ages to become (and stay) physically active, despite their limitations. **Everyone dances, even those in wheelchairs or using walkers or canes**. Jodie quickly discovered that the limitations that individuals with disabilities expe-

2 (http://www.essex.ac.uk/ces/esu/occasionalpapers/GreenExercise.pdf)

rience are generally placed on them by others. So, sign up for a class, or grab a few friends and head out for an evening, and see what develops – you may surprise yourself. Of course, you can always just crank up the tunes and bounce around at home – whatever it takes to get you inspired and moving.

Muscle Moves

Just as cardio has its benefits, so too does strength training. On a basic level, our bodies cannot perform a certain activity if we do not have enough muscle. At a more complex level, strength training involves using weights (including your own body) to build muscle mass and strength. Weights can include free weights, machines, resistance bands, or your own body. It may sound scary, but you will be surprised by your body's capacity – we assure you! Like cardio, strength training helps your body to burn calories, decrease pain, increase bone mass, and reduce stress, as well as increasing your ability to perform more complex cardio exercises. Unfortunately, as we age, muscle mass decreases and can be replaced with fat, and this same process can occur when you are sick and your body is retrieving energy from your muscles to help your body fight the illness.

As is the case with any activity, it is important to ensure proper technique to increase benefits and reduce the chance of injury while training with weights, and this is where physiotherapists or personal trainers can help. Weights can be done fast or slow, and with higher or lower loadings. It's always best to start slowly, with low weights, not only to give your body a chance to adjust to lifting weights, but also to learn the proper technique and "feel" of each movement. For more specific ideas and routines, speak to a physiotherapist or exercise professional/trainer, and/or check the Internet (with caution, of course). Make sure you listen to your body so that you can find the perfect balance between challenging yourself and overdoing things. Always remember that you are exercising to get healthier – not to get hurt!

Weight training can sometimes seem overwhelming, even scary – what if you hurt yourself, what if you are not doing it right, what if you look silly? Jodie faced all of these fears when she started doing strength training on a regular basis. Unfortunately, Jodie only began to lift weights regularly after being diagnosed with osteoporosis, likely as a result of years of steroid use (sound familiar?). She decided to seek advice from a personal trainer regarding what movements were safe and which were unsafe because of her reduced range of motion throughout her lower back, where the osteoporosis was located. To her surprise, she quickly became addicted to lifting weights, and now, whenever she gets busy and neglects her routine, her body lets her know by starting to ache. After a couple of years of careful exercise (both cardio and strength training), Jodie is happy to announce that her bone density is now back to normal. If that isn't great motivation, what is?!

As with cardio, there are numerous ways of increasing the degree of difficulty with strength training: (1) increase number of repetitions and/or weight; (2) lift weights at different angles; (3) lift increasingly higher or lower weights, with numerous repetitions, until you can't move any more (this is called pyramid work); (4) complete activities while jumping, or on an uneven surface (like a plank or Bosu™ ball); (5) work two different muscle groups at the same time; or (6) use your own body mass as resistance. The options are endless.

So, for all you weight-training newbies – give it a shot! **Our key word of advice: everyone else who is at the gym is concentrating on themselves, believe it or not**, and won't notice if you are only lifting a couple of pounds and/ or if you are pulling funny faces. You will be surprised just how far you can push yourself – sometimes literally!

Flex-ability

Stretching is an integral part of any exercise routine, as mentioned earlier, especially for preventing injuries. It is important to maintain a certain amount of flexibility, not only for fitness, but also for everyday life, and stretching can also help you to achieve this. There are a couple of important tips to keep in mind while stretching:

Tip #1: Do not stretch past your natural limit. You don't need to be touching your toes or bending your back as far as your instructor. Not everyone has the same level of flexibility. When stretching, you should only feel a slight pulling, and a minimal amount of pain – it should not be unbearable. Each stretch should be done 2–3 times and held for at least 15 seconds, without bouncing, with slow even breathing. Try to stretch a little further each time.

Tip #2: Modify stretches as needed. Just as with cardio and strength training activities, stretching can be modified to permit everyone to stretch relevant muscle groups. Jodie learned how to modify stretches, as needed, to relieve pressure on her lower back, due to her osteoporosis. These modifications included stretches for the abdominals, back, and legs, as a lot of the typical stretches for these areas involve bending. If you are not sure what your body can handle, please consult your lupus specialist, another specialist, and/or their affiliated physiotherapist. Once you have this information, a good personal trainer can show you modified versions of various exercises. This is invaluable information, as it will serve you well throughout your life, so we feel that paying for one session with a skilled personal trainer is well worth the investment. If you are already attending a training center, there are usually trainers roaming around the center who are there specifically to ensure that everyone is moving safely and correctly. Feel free to use this resource; for example, ask them how you can stretch your calf muscle without sitting on the floor and bending forward.

Tip #3: Stretching is not just for immediately before or after exercising. Stretching is meant to be a lifelong activity that will help you to maintain a certain level of fitness and flexibility. If you are unable to attend the gym on a regular basis, either because of time or financial constraints, or dipping energy levels, regular stretching is the very least you can do for your body. Think about it; by stretching, you keep your muscles and joints as flexible as possible, and maintains regular blood flow throughout your body. When someone is confined to hospital for any length of time, the two things the staff encourage are daily walks and daily stretching (the importance of walking has already been discussed). Because we now know that all stretches can be modified to fit your physical needs and current level of ability, there is no excuse. Stretching is exercise in itself: it's meditative, it's relaxing, and it's easy to incorporate into your daily routine. Some people prefer to do their stretches at the gym, while others prefer first thing in the morning or immediately before bed. Do whatever works best for you – as long as you stretch regularly. Just remember to warm up first!

Rest and Recovery

Although we have been stressing the importance of regular cardio and strength training activities, as well as stretching, it is equally important to give your body time to rest and recover. Do not use the same muscle groups two days in a row, and give your body at least one day of rest from intense cardio activity each week. And always listen to your body to determine whether additional rest days are required. Rest also includes getting adequate sleep, because the majority of your body's recovery will occur while you are sleeping. **Resting can be a form of meditation.** The most important component of meditation is focusing on your breathing, and forgetting about everything that is happening around you. Sometimes, meditation can be a means of focusing on something that is happening to you, in order to truly appreciate the experience. For example, focusing on your breathing during a difficult exercise session can serve as distraction, and may improve your performance.

Always Listen to Your Body

As important as exercise is in maintaining your health, there will be some days when you simply cannot bring yourself to exercise. Sometimes, the symptoms of your lupus flare-up will be too severe, in which case your priority should be to simply rest and let your body recover. Sometimes, you will simply be too exhausted. That's okay. Don't judge yourself or feel bad. Just relax, read a book or watch a movie, and go to bed early. When you feel better (and you *will* feel better), start up again with some light exercise. **Be sure to savor the pleasure of your moving body.** You might have lupus, but at least you're still here to experience the pleasure of your muscles moving, your heart beating, and your strong, steady breaths.

Get Motivated!

The main reasons why people don't stick to an exercise routine are that they get bored, or they feel that they no longer have enough time, so we want to give you a few ideas that will hopefully keep you active for the rest of your life. While we all feel super-excited to be starting a new routine, we are all at risk of eventually getting bored, and so we need ways to keep us as motivated as we were when we began our new healthy lifestyle.

Being motivated is the most important aspect of getting physically active, but maintaining your motivation is the hardest thing to achieve. When you are feeling sick and/or upset, it is really hard to find the drive to move your body. Often, with lupus, you just feel defeated – both physically and mentally. Sometimes, all you want to do (or can do) is lie down. This is completely normal. While it is entirely understandable that sometimes you are not motivated to do some exercise, you cannot let that stop you from moving your body as much as possible. When you are physically able to, it is crucial that you do *some* physical activity. You will feel so much better, it will keep you energized, and it may help you to heal more quickly. Although being motivated to do physical activity is hard, it is *not* impossible.

Just because you have one day when you're lacking motivation and can't bring yourself to do anything physically active, don't let this stop you from continuing on your fitness journey. Don't let a temporary lack of motivation get you down. It's important to realize that we all have "off" days. Be gentle with yourself. Don't think, "I missed today, so now I am a failure, and there is no sense in starting again tomorrow." Jump back into your routine as soon as you are able. Being motivated is a challenge, but this is your body, and you should do everything you can to keep it in as good working order as possible, and enjoy it! Get out there and move! Here are some tips to help get you through those days when you feel like staying on the couch.

1. **Enjoyment:** Choose activities that you enjoy doing to avoid getting bored and becoming unmotivated. We all know that it is much easier to do things that we actually like doing, and exercise is no different. If you enjoy walking, then be sure to take long walks! If you like turning up the music loud in your bedroom and rocking out, then go ahead and just do it! If you are not sure what you like, try all kinds of different activities until you find the one that you like best. Sometimes, enjoyment comes from doing an activity with a friend – an exercise buddy. This will be someone you can depend on to meet up with you for exercise on a regular basis. Most importantly, your buddy should be fun. They can help you to get and stay motivated. Jessica has two exercise buddies, and she has such a great time with them that exercise is not a chore at all, in fact she finds that the activity they do most of is laughing!

2. **Variety:** Trying different activities is important for several reasons. First, you need to find an activity that keeps you interested. Then, once you have found an activity that you enjoy, you need variety to keep you going mentally and physically. It is important to keep challenging your body with new activities to continue to get positive results. Don't be afraid to try new things. Find out what your friends are doing, and try something new together. Being active does not necessarily mean going to the gym or going for a walk every day. Get yourself moving in whatever way inspires you. One day you can do yoga, the next day a light run, the next day a hike in your favorite park, etc. Be creative (Dance Dance Revolution™ anyone?) and be daring. Try Tai Chi. Join a salsa class. Find or rent an exercise DVD that looks like fun. Play tennis on a Wii™. Go for a swim. Play Frisbee with your kids or friends. The options are endless.

3. **Timing:** We are all very busy, and it is even more difficult to find the time when you are trying to get enough sleep and balance your stress levels to avoid a lupus flare-up. However, just as we find time in our schedule to do laundry, it is important to find time to get some exercise. Just as we schedule visits to the doctor around our school/work commitments, we need to schedule our exercise time. Exercise is crucial to your mental and physical health, so dedicate some time to improving yourself, and protect that time from other commitments. It is much easier to maintain an exercise routine once it is part of your daily routine – just like taking a shower. If it is easier to do 20 minutes in the morning and 20 minutes in the evening (as opposed to 40 minutes in one chunk) that's fine. Find what works for you to ensure that you can fit in adequate exercise on a daily and weekly basis. Some people find it helpful to have their exercise time scheduled for them, such as joining classes that have a definite time and place for the activity. Going to a class will "force" you to make time to do the activities that you enjoy and get your body moving. If you are pressed for time, there are lots of ways to incorporate activity into your daily routine. For example, take the stairs instead of the elevator, or walk around while you're on the phone. In short, just try to move around whenever you can. This will make your body stronger, and keep you energized throughout the day.

4. **Exercise routine:** If you are uncertain about how much cardio, strength training, and stretching you require, one or two sessions with a personal trainer could be an invaluable investment. They should also provide you with tips regarding proper technique. A personal trainer will take into consideration your energy level, your best time of day to exercise, your current level of ability, your physical capacity, and your personal goals to help you put together a personal program. Some people find it helpful to have a weekly routine mapped out for them, instead of having to decide what activity they would like to do each day.

5. **Schedule:** Maintaining your routine during the holidays, exams, and other particularly busy periods of the year can be challenging. If it is not possible to keep to your usual days/hours, then simply modify your routine as required. Always remember though, the more exercise you get during these busy times, the more energy you will have, and fitting in some exercise will reduce your stress levels and your likelihood of getting sick. Consider your options carefully. If you only have one week of vacation, it might be best to simply enjoy it, so that you don't regret missing out. However, if your vacation time is more than one week, it might be best to continue to follow your routine as closely as possible for part of the time, while permitting yourself a few days off as a treat. Some people actually believe that taking one week off every few months is helpful to an exercise routine, while others believe that you should maintain a minimum level of exercise at all times, even if it is not at the same intensity as usual. The bottom line is, do what feels right for you, and understand that finding the right balance is something of a fine art.

6. **Pain:** There will be times when you are in so much pain that movement is simply not possible, but what about those times when you are still able to do some exercise? Try something less strenuous, like walking or swimming, or do some light and easy stretches (check out the section on Flexibility for ideas). Although pain is definitely a good reason to ease up on exercise, you don't have to give it up completely. Once again, be creative and be open to other activities that are light and fun. The activity may help to ease your pain and give your body some relief. Just do your best, and as always, pay attention to your body's needs.

For those of us with lupus, motivation-related barriers (those listed above) are not the only things that might hold us back from committing 100% to regular exercise. An additional barrier to exercise can be our sun sensitivity. While this is a concern, there are lots of exercises that are sun-safe. For instance, there are so many indoor activities available. Think about it; most people tend to do physical exercise indoors simply because it is too cold in the winter and too hot in the summer. Gyms and fitness classes are almost always indoors. Furthermore, you can take advantage of technology through options such as DVDs, online fitness programs, or even a Wii™. However, if you really love being outside and always exercising indoors seems like a bore to you, try working out in the early morning or late evening, when the effects of the sun are at their lowest. When exercising outdoors, be sure to wear plenty of sweatproof sunscreen, a hat, and light clothes that cover a large proportion of your body. Even though you may be sun-sensitive, you can still enjoy the boost from exercising outdoors.

Emotional Barriers?

Once you are diagnosed, exercising is a must in order to remain as healthy as possible, but what happens if you were already active prior to having this illness? How do you cope with changing your fitness routine and previous level of intensity? Those of us who were active prior to being diagnosed with lupus need to let go of some aspects of our former selves and create some new post-lupus fitness goals.

Jessica experienced this firsthand, and the first thing she had to do was "grieve" her former fitness self. Pre-lupus, Jessica was a bit of a gym rat. She loved to exercise, worked out almost every day, and even completed two half-marathons. All of her friends went to the gym daily as part of their social life, so when she began to get sick, a year before eventually being diagnosed with lupus, her previously extremely active life took a dramatic turn for the worse. Suddenly, she couldn't take deep breaths anymore (she had pleuritis), and had terrible pain in her joints (arthritis). She was always tired, and could no longer make it to the gym every day. This had a dramatic effect on her self-esteem, because she had taken great pride in her physical capabilities. Her social life was also affected, because her friends were still hanging out together at the gym without her. When she finally got diagnosed and began to get her lupus under control, she was able to be a bit more active, but it took a long time to recover her former physical capabilities, and it took an even longer time for her to come to terms with, and accept, her new lupus body.

Altering her fitness regime and accepting her new post-lupus exercise limitations was an incredible challenge for Jessica, and she really struggled to find new daily activities that were not as intense as her former routines. This opened her eyes to yoga, and once she discovered this new way to move her body, she never looked back. Although she still does the occasional intense workout (such as a fitness "boot camp" or a spinning class), she has really benefited from more gentle and relaxing workouts. She now embraces her new fitness regime, and feels great!

We all have to accept our post-lupus bodies, and we also need to embrace our post-lupus physical capabilities. **The key to accepting your new, post-lupus exercise regime is to know your limits.** Don't push yourself through barriers of pain and frustration simply because of your previous capabilities. Don't compare your current efforts with your past physical achievements. Focus on what you can accomplish today, and be open to new possibilities. Lupus may change your fitness goals, but you can still set realistic and challenging targets. Always remember that with lupus, you can still achieve your dreams; it's just that they may be slightly modified. Don't ever let lupus stop you from improving yourself. You can still reach your destination with a fit and healthy lupus body.

Just Do It

We hope that this chapter has inspired you to start moving or to explore a new and exciting activity. We are both devoted to moving our bodies, and thrive on the boost in energy that comes from regular exercise. However, we understand that lack of motivation is a huge barrier to regular physical activity. We also know that being organized is a very important way to eliminate many common excuses. So, try always having your workout gear ready to go, including a water bottle and your favorite, most energizing songs. There is always some time to exercise; you just need to find it and utilize it. Think about how much time you spend watching TV, or chatting online! Maybe you can decrease your screen time by 15 minutes and move your body instead.

And, don't forget to reward yourself for the milestones you achieve along your fitness journey! If you have a very low desire to exercise on some days, but you know that doing some exercise will surely benefit you, then set up a reward system. A reward can be watching your favorite TV show, reading a fun magazine, or painting your nails. Try not to use junk food as a reward, as that will counteract the benefits of your exercise. You should come to need rewards less and less as you adjust to your regular fitness routine, but they should still play a part in your healthy lifestyle. So, let your imagination fly, and see where your body's physical capabilities will take you!

Useful Sources of Information

Exercise Ideas
www.ideasforwomen.com
www.shapefit.com
www.mayoclinic.com
www.womensheartfoundation.org
www.shelterpub.com
www.womenshearts.org
www.learningmeditation.com
www.how-to-meditate.org
www.myfit.ca

Related Items
Parks Canada (www.pc.gc.ca)
Active Living Alliance for Canadians with Disabilities (ALACD)

HEALTHY EATING

Eating Well – Why Bother?

When you have lupus, there are many things that you cannot control (sunlight intensity, side effects from your medications, your next flare-up, etc.), but what you eat is not one of those things. You (for the most part) decide what you eat, and eating well will make a huge difference to your health. But eating well is not always easy, in fact it can be one of the hardest things to do! Whether they have lupus or not, most people struggle with healthy eating from time to time (or all the time!). So, don't worry if you feel that eating a balanced diet can sometimes be tough. There are several real obstacles to overcome when it comes to eating well when you have lupus. These include motivating yourself to eat well, knowing what food is healthy, planning meals, shopping for ingredients, cooking, and being too busy and/or sick to plan, shop, and cook. Although these challenges exist, they must be dealt with, because eating well is the cornerstone of being healthy.

If you have a chronic illness like lupus, eating well is absolutely crucial for managing your illness. You need lots of nutrients to keep your body healthy and strong! Helping your body to function better with proper nutrition will really help you deal with the rest of the problems associated with the illness. Here are some important reasons why eating a balanced diet is key for those with lupus:

1. A balanced diet will help you achieve and maintain a healthy weight – Weight management is extremely important in managing lupus and optimizing your health. One of the most common side effects of the main medication that is prescribed to treat lupus (prednisone) is weight gain. Being overweight is generally not good for your overall health, and gaining a lot of weight can place unnecessary strain on our joints and organs. Eating healthy foods and watching portion sizes are the most important components of weight management.

2. Healthy eating can strengthen your immune system – Eating nutritious meals can improve your immune system. Your body needs lots of nutrients in order to be strong and to fight illnesses and stressors, especially lupus and the medications that are used to treat it. Having a top-notch immune system can stop minor illnesses (such as colds or infections) from becoming a more serious problem.

3. Eating well gives you more energy – Getting lots of nutrients in your diet will give you more energy! Your body will function better, and you won't feel as sluggish all of the time. Not having enough energy to do even simple tasks is a major problem for those of us with lupus. Eating healthy food can give you back some of that energy.

4. Healthy eating keeps your organs healthy –When you have lupus, having efficient and functioning organs is essential to your overall physical health. Many of the medications that we take can sometimes negatively impact our heart, lungs, brain, and other organs, so we need to counteract these effects with healthy food. You don't want to clog up the system with too much junk. Your organs are already working very hard to process all the medication you take to stay healthy. Do everything you can to keep your body systems "clean"!

5. Healthy eating reduces the risk of (pretty much) every other illness – Research has shown that a healthy diet is key in preventing almost all other chronic health conditions. Having lupus is hard enough, so it is important to do our best to reduce our chances of developing other health complications.

What Does It Mean to Eat Well?

But what does eating well really mean? And how do you do it? **The key to eating well is balance**, but this simple statement can actually get quite confusing, because there is so much information about food and dieting out there. Some of the information is good and reasonable, some of it is false, and some of it is downright dangerous. When you have a condition like lupus, you have to be even more careful about what (and how much) you put into your body. Therefore, it is super important that you consult a doctor or nutritionist/ registered dietician about your dietary needs. In Canada, you can find one at www.dietitians.ca (this website also has lots of information about nutritious diets), but no matter where you live, you can always ask your doctor for a refer- ral and/or find credible websites that will provide information on where to find dieticians or about healthy eating.

There are also lots of resources out there such as books, magazines, and websites. This is great, but you have to be careful and selective about the information that is provided. **Always talk to your doctor and/or a registered dietician/nutritionist about your nutritional choices and concerns.** Use your instincts and common sense. If something sounds too good to be true (like an all-bacon diet), it probably is.

Healthy vs. unhealthy

Most of us know what foods are really good for us (fruit, veggies) and what foods are not so good for us (cookies, fries). The main idea is to eat more of the healthy foods and less of the unhealthy foods. Avoiding them completely is kind of unrealistic, and could result in you binge eating at a later point as a result of feeling deprived. Eating unhealthy foods is very tempting, especially in North America, where fatty, salty, and sugary foods are so readily available (there seems to be a fast food restaurant on every corner!). To eat well, we need to focus on eating plenty of fruit, vegetables, lean protein sources (fish, chicken, tofu), and healthy carbohydrate choices (whole wheat pasta/rice), and only rarely succumb to the temptation of less healthy choices. The reason why you should try to eat healthy foods every day is because these foods have tons of nutrients, which is what you need not only to survive, but also to thrive. Un- healthy foods tend to have less of these crucial nutrients that your body needs to not only heal, but also to perform everyday activities. Unhealthy foods also tend to include other ingredients that can cause harm to your body if you ingest too much of them. Avoiding unhealthy food is challenging, because it is really appealing and everywhere. Therefore, it is best to develop some strategies to reduce your consumption of "junk food." The best strategy is to make sure that your fridge and pantry are both filled with healthy foods, and that unhealthy foods don't even make it inside your door. **Try not to buy unhealthy food in the first place!** Another way to avoid eating too much unhealthy food is to limit yourself to one treat each day (for example, Jessica has a piece of dark chocolate every day). That way, you won't feel like you're missing out and over-indulge later. Take a packed lunch to work/school, so that you won't be tempted by the fries in the cafeteria. When you go out driving, pack some healthy snacks (carrot sticks, fruit, nuts, etc.) so that you are not tempted to purchase fast food when you stop for gas. Carry a water bottle with you wherever you go to avoid buying sugary soft drinks or juices – it's better to help you stay hydrated, and cheaper too! It can be tough to (mostly) always eat healthy, but do your best!

Natural vs. processed

Another way to approach healthy eating is to eat foods that are as close as possible to their "natural" state and avoid "fake" and overly processed foods. For example, fresh fruit and vegetables are ready for consumption, and have absolutely no added ingredients. Compare that with store-bought chips and cookies (even crackers), and pre-made foods such as lasagnas or frozen dinners. Usually, these processed, packaged foods contain numerous additional ingredients that contain far more calories, salt, sugar, and fat than natural foods. Many of these "extras" are added to processed food to provide color and flavor, and to ensure that the product can last for a longer time on the shelf. It is very important to read the list of ingredients contained in every product that you consume. You may be shocked to learn what's in your food! You may not even know what the ingredients are (maybe you can't even pronounce them!). So, do your best to eat mostly fresh food. One great option for healthy, natural foods is to check out your local farmers market. However, don't get too hung up on the need to eat 'organic' food. There are limited guidelines regarding what foods are able to be labeled as 'organic,' and some of these choices may not be quite as healthy as you think! You can do some research about organic foods at www.eatrightontario.ca/en/viewdocument.aspx?id=452. Be careful of meat substitutes produced for vegetarians too, because these can be just as unhealthy as processed meat products. Do a bit of research and read labels.

Portion control

It's not just what you eat, but how much, so it is worth looking into proper serving sizes. Although, it is very important to eat healthy food for its nutritional content, if you want to either lose, gain, or maintain body weight, you need to consider both the serving sizes and the calorie numbers. This also applies to what you drink. It is very important to drink as much water as possible, and to think about the calories included in each juice, soda pop, or frappucino™ that you consume. These are calories that most individuals forget to include in their portion control!

Prior to her diagnosis, Jessica was for the most part eating a pretty healthy and balanced diet, but after her diagnosis, she sought guidance because she was taking prednisone, and did not want to gain too much weight. She consulted a registered dietician, who taught her how to determine appropriate portion sizes. Did you know that one serving of protein should be the size of a deck of cards? Or that one serving of carbohydrates should be ½ cup, or just one slice of bread? Another strategy is to make sure that at least half of your plate is filled with veggies. Then, one quarter of your plate can contain protein, while the other quarter can contain carbohydrates. Another trick that Jessica has used to help her find the right portion sizes is to simply use smaller plates (if you are trying to maintain or lose weight, this is a great, easy, and low-cost solution). Paying attention to her portion sizes helped Jessica to lose some of the "prednisone weight" that she had gained. Her dietician really helped her understand serving sizes, and to learn how to "eyeball" the required amounts of various food types that she needed, so she highly recommends seeking the help of a dietician.

But, But, But...Barriers

We all know that we should be eating healthy food almost all of the time. However, there are several obstacles that can prevent those of us with lupus from eating well. We need to know how we can overcome those obstacles.

Obstacle #1: Lack of motivation

The hardest part, of course, is being motivated to eat well, especially when you are dealing with an illness like lupus. It can be very difficult to continually encourage yourself to eat well all the time. Having lupus is hard enough, and so striving for healthy eating can easily fall by the wayside, especially when you're dealing with a major flare-up, or in pain, or constantly tired. Sometimes, just getting out of bed can be tough enough, so who cares about healthy eating!? It is entirely understandable that eating nutritious meals may not register on your radar, and that eating well doesn't seem important when you have what feel like bigger problems to deal with. However, **healthy eating will actually help you manage your lupus symptoms**, and give you the energy to tackle other tasks in your life. When you eat well, you will be absorbing nutrients that will make you healthier, give you more energy, and help you to heal, so it is worth making the effort to eat a range of fresh vegetables, fruits, whole grains, lean proteins and low-fat dairy. You will feel so much better, and your lupus will likely get better too.

Obstacle #2: Being too sick

This is a definite concern, because at some point all of us with lupus will have to deal with a major flare-up. It is hard to plan and prepare healthy meals every day when you are healthy, let alone when you are feeling really sick. This is when you call up your "assistants." Don't be afraid to ask your family and friends for help. Perhaps they can come over (if you don't live with them) and help you prepare healthy meals. Once the food has been prepared, it can be frozen in meal-size portions, so all you need to do is heat and serve. Or perhaps someone can get you some groceries. If your family and friends are unavailable, many stores offer online grocery shopping and home delivery. **The key is to not be afraid to ask for help.** When you are really ill, your first priority should be to get better, not be the perfect cook. On the other hand, when you are really ill, eating well will help to speed up your recovery, because you will be feeding your body the nutrients it needs to get better. A meal doesn't need to be complicated to be nutritious. Here is a list of some easy and healthy meal options:

- Sandwiches
- Salads
- Stir-fries
- Pastas
- Smoothies
- Soups

Here are a few other tips to help you along: (1) take advantage of frozen fruits, veggies, and meats, as well as a few healthy frozen meals (just make sure you read the labels carefully); (2) Try some of the many healthy ready-made meals that are available; and (3) don't be afraid of laborsaving devices, like food processors, blenders, and slow cookers. These devices are extremely useful when you are experiencing arthritis in your joints, or other lupus symptoms that limit your physical abilities in the kitchen. While you are healthy, do some research (Internet, magazines, cookbooks) and build up a file of recipes for simple, healthy meals that you can turn to when you get sick.

Obstacle #3: Lack of time

Not having the time to properly plan and cook nutritious meals is a common problem for many people. **They key is to plan your time and meals as best you can.** The first step is to make sure you have all the necessary ingredients at the ready. It's very important to have a stock of the basics in your kitchen. The basics will be different for everyone, but it's important to know the core ingredients of the meals that you eat regularly. In addition, many people plan

FABULUPUS

their meals for the week ahead, which enables them to finalize their grocery list and make full, economical use of ingredients, cut down on preparation time, and avoid the stress of having to think up a new meal each day. For example, you might fry some vegetables for tacos on Monday, and then add the leftover vegetables to some pasta on Tuesday. You should also plan your breakfasts, lunches, and snacks, to avoid the temptation of fast food. You can record all your meals on a calendar (electronic or paper), or simply keep a list. If this all seems a little too intense for you, just try to have a rough idea of some healthy meals that you can pull together. Make sure that you incorporate some flexibility, because as you know, there are always unexpected twists and turns in your life. When you have at least some idea of the meals you want to make during the coming week, you can purchase all your groceries (either by going shopping in a store if you're up to it, or online if you're not) that you will need in one hit. This ensures that you will have all your ingredients at your fingertips so that you don't have to scrounge around looking for substitute items, and won't have to spend precious time and energy making emergency runs to the grocery store. Sometimes it can be fun to look at what food is on sale for the week, and then plan your meals with those items in mind. This is a great way to incorporate new, healthy foods into your diet, and save a little money at the same time!

Another tip is to make some time (such as on the weekend or when you have an evening free) to prepare several meals in advance by cooking in bulk (it doesn't take much more time to cook a six-serve casserole than it takes to cook a single serve) and then freezing the food in meal-sized portions. Then, all you have to do when the time comes to enjoy them is heat and eat. Jessica stocks up on fruits and veggies every week and eats those as snacks (it's easy, fast, and nutritious), while Jodie always makes her lunches the night before while watching her favorite television shows. Try different strategies to see what works best for you.

Obstacle #4: You don't like to cook

Cooking may seem like a drag to many people who view it as just

102

another chore that they have to do. Jessica completely understands this, because she has a love/hate relationship with cooking. Her goal is to keep things as simple as possible, but she also likes to learn new things. If you don't like cooking, then don't put unnecessary stress on yourself thinking that you have to become a gourmet cook. However, you do need to learn to prepare most of your meals, as this is likely to be both the healthiest and cheapest way to eat. **Cooking does not have to be hard!** Indeed, in some ways, the simple, repetitive acts of stirring sauces or cutting vegetables can actually become a meditation, and can help to ease stress! Ask someone to teach you the basics, or buy/borrow some cookbooks. There are plenty that specialize in simple, delicious, healthy and easy-to-prepare meals. There are also many grocery stores, local community centers, and colleges that offer basic cooking classes where you can learn new techniques and meet new friends. Don't be afraid of experimenting with new ways to cook, or trying new varieties of food (have you ever made Pho at home?). You may even discover a whole new side to yourself; maybe there is a brilliant cook hidden inside you, just waiting to be let loose!

Obstacle #5: Living at home with your parents

When you live at home with your parents, what you eat may not necessarily be totally up to you. This lack of control can be very frustrating, and sometimes overwhelming. Hopefully, your parents/caregivers often eat healthy meals, and respect your need/desire to eat properly. However, if they don't, then it's up to you to take the initiative and try to change your diet for the better. If you have siblings, ask for their help in changing your family's eating habits. The best thing to do is to approach your parents/guardians in a calm way, and explain to them why it's really important that you eat well. You can also enlist the help of your doctor or dietician. If your parents still accompany you to your medical appointments, you can ask your medical team to talk with them about the importance of eating nutritious, well-balanced meals. This might help to motivate your parents to try to improve the family's nutrition. Even if your parents don't come to your appointments with you, your doctor or dietician can give you some information pamphlets that you can bring home and share with your family. Otherwise, you can seek the help of a registered dietician, who will be able to give you some strategies on how to eat as well as possible, while respecting your family's wish not to join you. Although it might be tempting to eat unhealthy food, you have to fight this urge, because your overall health and ability to manage your condition depends on your healthy eating. Taking charge of your diet will also help you take charge of your lupus. This is something you simply cannot ignore!

Obstacle #6: Lack of money

If you are a student, or unable to work, concerns about money are an ever-present reality, and spending money on nutritious food may seem like an outrageous expense. Yet, healthy eating is the key to being healthy overall! So, you need to find creative ways to eat well on a budget. The first thing is to have a realistic food budget, and to make sure you are buying enough food to get all the nutrients you need. Once you have a budget, make a list of the healthy foods that you need, and stick to the list when you go into grocery stores. This will help you to resist the temptation to buy more than you need, or to buy unhealthy food. There are several ways to save money on food: (a) go to discount grocery stores, because these places sell pretty good produce (fruits and vegetables) for a lower price; (b) buy staples, such as rice and pasta, at bulk food stores; (c) buy fruits and veggies when they are in season; (d) go to local farmers' markets for in-season fruits, veggies, and locally produced meat and bread; and (e) use coupons and check weekly pamphlets for sales. The main idea is to stick to your budget and prioritize buying natural and whole foods.

It may seem like unhealthy food (such as fast food or junk food) is cheaper, but **eating out actually costs more than preparing meals at home, and will also cost you your health in the long run.** The price you pay in terms of your health is simply not worth it! Therefore, you need to invest in your health by doing your best to consume fresh, healthy food that is rich in nutrients and vitamins.

Start Today!

It is never too late (or too early) to start eating well. There are lots of reasons why you should do it, and lots of resources out there to help you get started, and to stick with it. **Once you start to eat better, you will start to feel better, and you will be even more motivated to stick with your new food choices.** Start small, with some achievable goals, like to eat an apple a day, or to stop eating fries for lunch every day. Don't give up. You can still incorporate some treats into your diet; you just can't eat junk all the time. Your body needs the nutrients and vitamins that only a well-rounded diet can provide. Once you are used to eating well most of the time, you will notice a difference in how your body feels after eating a less healthy meal. Jodie still loves sharing a plate of nachos with a friend, but hates how she feels afterwards (tired, bloated, and less energetic at the gym). Noticing how her body responds to eating well compared with how it responds to unhealthy eating really motivates Jodie to keep eating well (most of the time).

If you have lupus, it is even more important that your body gets the right amount of nutrients, vitamins, and calories it needs to stay strong and healthy, in addition to giving you the strength and energy that you need to manage your condition. Don't delay for one more day, or say you'll start tomorrow. Start now, and get a head start on feeling better and managing your illness!

SELF-ESTEEM & STYLE

Lupus and Your Self

Self-esteem is about how much or how little you believe you are worth. Being diagnosed and living with lupus can make you feel worthless. Even if you had healthy self-esteem before you found out you had lupus, it can still decline after you are diagnosed. If you were already struggling with your self-worth, then lupus can certainly add another downer to your perception. This chapter is about not only understanding how having lupus can make you feel bad about yourself, but also about how you can learn to feel great. We hope we can help you to think of yourself in a new, brighter light!

How does lupus bring down your self-esteem, and how can you bring it back up? Lupus can affect your self-esteem in many ways. First, as lupus is an illness, being diagnosed automatically means that your body is not totally healthy, and this fact alone can have a terrible impact on your self-image. Being and feeling healthy is a huge part of how people view themselves. Being diagnosed with lupus can come as a big shock for people who thought they were healthy, and would continue to be healthy for a long time to come. You are likely also feeling terribly sick, which can also contribute to not feeling good about yourself. Just as your body needs time to heal, you also need to give your mind time to adjust and "heal." You will need to learn to gradually accept that you have lupus, what that means for your life, and what that means for who you think you are as a person. Always remember that you are not your lupus, and that there is so much more to you and your life. You can use this experience to grow stronger, to appreciate your strengths, and to move forward with what is important in your life. It's not easy, but you can do this! It is important to always remember that having lupus does not define you as a person. It is just one part of you, and you can use this experience to grow and become even more positive, creative, successful, and loving.

Second, the unpredictability of lupus can make developing and maintaining a healthy sense of self-esteem a huge challenge. Because another flare-up can strike at any time, the uncertainty can make it harder for you to truly develop a good sense of worth. You can also expect that your self-esteem will suffer every time you have a flare-up. This is tough, because you have to constantly keep pumping yourself up and building up your self-esteem. However, know that each time you work on yourself, you will get stronger and stronger. It will gradually get easier, and you will also get better at identifying what is important in your life, and what helps you to stay positive about yourself.

Third, lupus can affect your self-image by draining you of your energy and zest for life. You may often feel weak and sick, and can end up thinking that you are useless, and that you can't accomplish anything anymore. This can be damaging to your self-image, especially if you were used to having lots of energy and being able to accomplish lots of things before you were diagnosed. However, once the lupus is under control, you will feel so much better, and your energy will start to come back. In the meantime, you need to learn to manage your energy, and this process can help you to realize what is truly important in your life (see the Stress & Energy chapter for suggestions). There are also lots of suggestions on ways to boost your energy in that chapter. Once you start accomplishing a few things, you will gain an even greater appreciation for yourself. Your self-esteem will improve, because you were able to do all those things and still manage your chronic illness!

Fourth, one of the most dramatic ways in which lupus can affect your self-esteem is through changes to your body. Our body image is very much linked to our self-esteem. One of the most common complaints from people with lupus is weight gain due to medication side effects or decreased physical activity due to pain and/or fatigue. Once you start to feel like you have gained weight, your self-esteem can plummet, as can your energy, which only leads you to feel more lazy and worthless. It can be a vicious cycle! Weight gain can be very hard on teenagers and young adults, because our society is constantly sending the message that thinner is better (which is not necessarily the truth!).

You may also compare yourself to your friends, who are not gaining weight like you, and are not dealing with a chronic illness like you. In reality, almost everyone struggles with his or her weight at one time or another. Jessica gained weight when she started taking prednisone, which made her feel really terrible, because her wedding day was approaching. First, she had to accept the fact that she had gained weight, and that this was due to medication that she was taking to control her illness. Then, she realized that she needed to be proactive by eating as well as she could and exercising to keep fit. Now, Jessica looks back on her wedding day (and photos) and is glad that she was not overly obsessed with her looks, and that she really enjoyed the big day. She was still a beautiful bride!

In addition to weight gain, there are other ways in which your body may change with lupus that might affect your self-image. These include weight loss, rashes, hair changes, and physical disability.

Weight loss

Sometimes when you are becoming ill with a flare-up, you actually start to lose weight, and can even become very thin, which can be quite dangerous. The first thing to do is to contact your doctor. It can be quite tempting to not do anything about weight loss (especially at first, when people may be complimenting you), but this can be an important alarm bell telling you that a flare-up is starting. Any weight changes should be reported to your doctor immediately. You may need some additional medication, and/or to gain some weight. Of course, if you need to gain weight, you should speak to a registered dietician for advice on how to do so in a healthy way.

If you've lost some weight and are feeling self-conscious about it, you can use clothes to make yourself feel better (see the Style Tips section later in this chapter). Most importantly, though, you shouldn't focus too much on your weight loss. There is so much more to you and your life than how much you weigh. Even though you may be getting compliments about your weight loss, especially because our society values a certain body type, always be mindful of how your weight changes affect your self-esteem, because your weight shouldn't be the only factor contributing to how you feel about yourself!

Skin rashes

The recurring "butterfly" rash is quite a common aspect of lupus, and it often appears on the face, making it hard to hide. People often ask insensitive questions, which can be really embarrassing and very tough to deal with. You might feel like you want to stop going out so that you can avoid seeing people and having to face their stares and questions, but it's best to try and accept your rash, and how others react to it, and continue to live your life as normally as possible. It is through living normally that you will stay connected to what is important to you, and that is what will keep your self-esteem high. If you are really self-conscious about your rashes, there are various cosmetics that you can use to minimize the appearance. As always, talk to your doctor and/or dermatologist if you notice any changes, or want prescription assistance with coverage. And always keep in mind that the rash is not permanent, and will eventually settle, and possibly even disappear, in time.

Hair changes

A rather common and fairly devastating effect of lupus is alopecia, or hair loss. It is an awful feeling when you brush your hair and clumps come right off your head. Although this is hard to accept, trust us, it will get better. This hair loss is temporary, and your hair will eventually grow back. In the meantime, there are options such as adopting a shorter hairstyle that will create the impression of greater hair thickness. Coloring your hair might also help. Depending on the severity of the hair loss, you might think about wearing hats, scarves, and/or wigs – get creative! Although it is very difficult to live with thinning hair, do not despair, and try not to hide! Hiding and spending time alone will only lead to you feeling more down, because you will not be living your normal life. Remember, you have an illness from which you will eventually recover. In the meantime, you need to keep your spirits up!

Physical disability

One particularly unfair aspect of lupus is the possibility of developing a physical disability. This can range from a crooked finger due to severe arthritis to needing special equipment to assist with your mobility. No matter what, it is a visible reminder to you and everyone you meet that you are different. It can take time to get used to your new body, and the physical limitations that come from having a disability, but a disability can also help you to really appreciate the other things that your body can do (see the Staying Active chapter). A disability can also help you to focus on what is important to you, your sense of self, and your quality of life. No matter what activities you want to continue with, challenge yourself to continue to participate, and strive to find the equipment you need to support you!

As for your social life, a physical disability can also help you to realize who your true friends are, because some people have a hard time hanging out with someone who looks different. Having said that, it can be hard to live with an "invisible" disability, because people find it difficult to believe that you have any limitations. In any case, the most important thing is for you to be true to yourself, take comfort from those who support you, continue to push boundaries to achieve your goals, and keep smiling – because you are fabulous!

Style Tips

No matter whether your physical change is weight gain or loss, or a physical disability, sometimes you will feel like dressing in such a way as to draw attention to yourself, while at other times you will want to hide as much as possible. Dressing appropriately in clothes that fit you well can have a huge positive effect on how you feel, and your self-image. Of course, when you are sick, you do not always feel like shopping, and you do not always have the energy. Likewise, you may not have the money to buy new clothes after having to spend money on illness-related stuff, and it can be challenging trying to keep up when your body is always changing! Here are a few tips that we have found helpful over our years of living with lupus. These tips take into consideration all the body-related issues we have discussed that can become an issue when you're living with lupus.

Here are few 'Dos' and 'Don'ts' that we want to share with you based on our experiences:

Don't be afraid to try wearing different styles and colors.

Don't ever be embarrassed or ashamed by your body type – everyone is different and beautiful!

Don't worry if your body shape is changing a bit due to medication or flare-up (or for any other reason) and just focus on finding clothes that fit and flatter your current shape.

Don't go shopping when you are feeling ill or uncomfortable.

Don't be pressured to buy something that you are not comfortable wearing.

Don't buy clothes/jewelry just to impress others. Buy the things that you like and that are within your budget.

Don't compare your body and style to other people. Remember that you have your own personal sense of style and it's fabulous!

Don't worry about trying to keep up with the latest fashions if they obviously don't suit your current body shape.

Don't worry if you can't fit into something that used to fit (even if it was just a few days ago); every day, your body might be a bit different. Only wear what is comfortable and flattering.

Don't forget to take a supportive friend/family member with you when you need extra advice

Don't be afraid to have your own personal look! Wear what you like and enjoy!

Do have comfortable, stylish clothes in different sizes and in both looser and tighter styles.

Do think 'softly contoured' when looking for the right fit.

Do find a good tailor – almost any garment can be altered to suit your specific shape

Do experiment with different looks to see what works best for you.

Do try and see if you enjoy shopping online (if you don't feel like trying anything on).

Do make sure to stay on budget and make sure you understand the return policy (both in real and virtual stores).

Do invest in a few key pieces, like a great coat, that make you feel good and go with many outfits. Having a few wonderful items will always make you feel good and nicely presented, even if you are not feeling all that great.

Do accessorize, and try different types of jewelry, scarves, and hats. Accessories complete any outfit, help to express your individuality, and focus attention where you want it (or away from where you don't want it). Accessories are also cheaper to replace if you want to change your look, rather than changing your key investment pieces.

Do wear hats, because not only do they cover your face, but they look good too! For maximal sun protection and fashion savvy, choose a dense material and a brim that is greater than 8 cm (or 3 inches).

Do invest in a quality (and stylish) pair of sunglasses. Larger-framed sunglasses can help protect your face from the sun's rays. Read the labels to ensure adequate UV protection.

Do investigate clothes with SPF protection if you are very sun-sensitive.

Do wear longer skirts, Capri pants, sleek knee-length shorts (Bermuda shorts) and long (or 3/4 length)-sleeved shirts in the summer to protect you from the sun.

Do make sure to have very warm, high-quality mitts (there are specialized mitts if you have Raynaud's) and very warm, high-quality boots for the winter.

Do be fabulous!

Overall, the key to maintaining a healthy image when you have lupus is to accept the changes to your body (as much as possible), and to then be proactive in dealing with them (check out the Healthy Eating and Staying Active chapters for lots of suggestions). Try not to despair; try to focus on all the positive things about yourself. You don't need to hide yourself; you should continue to do the things you love! Do things that make you feel good! You will always be beautiful, no matter how your lupus changes your body. Always remember that.

Be Fabulupus!

Healthy self-esteem doesn't just appear out of nowhere – you have to work on it! You have to actively try to bolster your self-esteem. Moreover, you have to do it as often as you can. Here are some tips to help you increase your self-esteem:

• Find a few positive affirmation statements (for instance, "I am strong", "I am healthy and happy", "I am calm") that really mean something to you, and repeat them to yourself regularly, either silently or out loud
• Write down positive thoughts every day (or as often as you can manage)
• Keep a journal of motivational quotes, and read it whenever you're feeling down
• Read uplifting books and/or articles
• Surround yourself with positive and motivating people (and stay away from those who don't make you feel good about yourself)
• Do activities that make you feel good!
• Find positive role models
• Try new things and new challenges. Accomplishments really boost your self-esteem!

LEISURE & TRAVEL

Give Me a Break!

Life is tough when you have lupus, so it's very important that you still have some fun, get out and about, and take some breaks from the obligations in your life. It is very easy to let thoughts about your illness take over your life, and although it can seem comforting to wallow in pity for a while, it is not a good coping strategy in the long term. You can also get bogged down by regular daily activities (such as school/work and/or chores), because they are harder and more time-consuming when you have lupus. It can be hard to make "downtime" a priority for healthy living. However, having fun and creating temporary escapes is essential to your long-term health, especially when you have a chronic health condition. That said, you still need to deal with your life, which includes your illness. You can't ignore your challenges permanently. Having fun is a fine balance between having enough of a distraction to enjoy a moment, while not overdoing it and putting yourself at risk of a flare-up. Even though you have lupus, you can still enjoy your life. The key is to live a balanced life. **Doing things that make you happy will help you cope with your illness** by reminding you about the good things life has to offer, rather than focusing on the limitations that your illness may impose. So go ahead and create a fabulous social life, participate in leisure activities, travel and explore! You can live life to the fullest!

Social Life

At times, it can seem like having any kind of social life (especially when you are experiencing a flare-up) is impossible. Jessica is a very sociable person, but the year before she was diagnosed, she was so sick that going out with friends was too exhausting, although she had no idea why. She couldn't participate in her regular activities with her friends, and she couldn't offer any explanation to them. Luckily, her friends not only understood, but also stood by her. Your friends/family may surprise you with how supportive they will be in relation to your new limitations. You may also be surprised at how creative you can be in finding ways that enable you to continue to engage in social activities whenever you are experiencing a flare-up.

Sure, there will be times when your social life won't be all that great. Please take comfort from knowing that these ups/downs in your social life are normal, even for those without a chronic health condition. That said, it is harder when you have lupus because the flare-ups can be so unpredictable. You may be planning on going to a really fun event, and then your lupus gets in the way, and you end up not being able to go. This can make you feel like you have no control, that your lupus is ruining your life, and that life is passing you by. This can also make you feel jealous of people who don't have lupus, because it seems like they get to have all the fun. These are all normal feelings. But you will soon learn to accept that you won't be able to make every party, or hang out with your friends all the time. Focus on your health first, because you can always have fun! There will be many, many more parties to go to in the future. If your friends are truly your friends, they will understand and help you to get through this tough time. They will be flexible with their plans, and will think of activities that you can share with them. If your friends are not support-ive, then they are not the kind of friends that you want in your life. These kinds of "friends" are negative influences, and will only cause your emotional and physical health to suffer. Take a deep breath, think of something positive, relax, and don't feel bad if you can't make it to every single party. You *will* get better, and you will get many chances to be the social butterfly that you are.

Like we said earlier in this chapter, even if you are experiencing a flare-up, you can still find ways to hang out with your friends. The options may depend on your health. If you are in the hospital, and you are comfortable with this, see if your friends can come visit you. If you need to stay at home and/or have a disability that makes going out all the time difficult, have your friends come over for a visit. Watch a movie, play games, or just chat. You don't have to isolate yourself just because you are ill. Remember that the good thing about lupus is that it is not contagious, so try to see people! If you are feeling well enough to go out, arrange activities that aren't a big drain on your energy, like going to a movie or meeting for coffee or a meal. Eventually, your flare-up will pass and you can return to your normal activities (going for a walk with a friend, or dancing all night long). **Although it is hard to plan things when you are not feeling well, if seeing your friends makes you feel better, try to schedule them in!** This can only benefit your overall health. Don't focus on the things you can't do, but focus on the things you *can* do.

Living at home with your parents/guardians can also be a challenge to maintaining your social life. They may feel overprotective when you are experiencing a flare-up, insisting that you rest all the time. You may need to tell your parents that it's important you get a chance to do the activities that you enjoy. This may be a hard message to present to your parents on your own, so see if someone on your rheumatology team can help bring this issue up at your next doctor's appointment. If your parents are reluctant because they are worried that having a social life will tire you out, see if they would be willing to compromise and allow you to try some low-key activities with your friends. For example, your friends can come over to your place to hang out. Start with some short visits. Once your parents see that being with your friends makes you happy, and that it is helping you to get through the flare-up, they may be more willing to discuss a wider range of activities.

Another challenge is maintaining your social life when you have a disability. You will need to do some research on places to hang out that are easily accessible. We talk about some options in the Staying Active chapter, so check it out for more details. Most importantly, make sure you stay connected with your friends. Seriously, it's important to have fun and not let lupus get you down – it just takes some extra creativity and organization.

Leisure Life

What exactly are "leisure" activities, and why are they important when you have lupus? Leisure time is basically time spent *not* working, but rather doing something *only* for pleasure (so no chores!). Leisure activities include reading, photography, yoga, writing, dancing, knitting, hiking, sports, playing an instrument, gardening, and the list goes on and on and on! **It's important to incorporate some leisure time into your life when you have lupus, because it gives you a much-needed break from constantly worrying about your illness.** You need a chance to unwind and relax by doing something (anything, really) that has nothing to do with your lupus or other obligations. As stress is a major trigger for increasing lupus symptoms, leisure activities can help you recover if you are experiencing a flare-up, and then help prevent another flare-up from occurring. Having hobbies in your life isn't silly or a waste of time – they can really help you manage your illness. Having some leisure in your life will make your lupus easier to manage, but the hard part can be actually doing activities!

There are potentially lots of barriers that can stop you from doing the things you love, but there are also lots of options to help you overcome these barriers. If you've already got activities that you like to do and you are still able to do them, that's awesome. Keep them up! However, sometimes this may be easier said than done. For example, as we mentioned earlier, before being diagnosed with lupus Jessica was an avid runner (she even completed two half-marathons), but after she was diagnosed with lupus she scaled back her running to ease the pressure on her joints. Now, she now takes long walks instead, which gives her the same sense of peace and accomplishment. Since learning to manage her lupus, now that she is feeling better, she has started to do some short runs on certain days to get a jolt of energy. You may also need to adjust how you manage your favorite activity, or change the activity altogether. Nonetheless, **it is completely normal to feel angry, frustrated, sad, and resentful that you have to give up something you enjoy so much.** It's tough to have to change something you really like when you have an illness. However, being flexible is key, and you will be able to find alternative activities that you will find equally enjoyable. For example, if you were really into scuba diving, then depending on your illness, you may have to stop scuba diving completely and do snorkeling instead. Sometimes, you may need to use special equipment to make it physically possible for you to continue participating in a particular activity. Using medical equipment can be embarrassing, but it can also be uplifting to do the things you enjoy, and to be independent!

However, sometimes having lupus means that you need to give up your favorite activity completely. For example, if you were an avid painter before being diagnosed with lupus, but now your joints are just too painful to even hold a brush, this change can be devastating. Take some time to mourn this loss, but then try to find something else to do! We all enjoy numerous activities in life, so shift your focus to something else. Maybe you'll find something to do that is related, like using computer programs to create or learn about art history, or taking virtual tours of art galleries online. Or maybe you'll try something completely different! Keep trying to find new hobbies and new things to do. Maybe you'll discover something you come to love even more than your original hobby!

If you currently don't have any hobbies, then start looking for some. Even though you have lupus, that doesn't mean that you have to stop enjoying yourself and your life. The most important criterion for your new leisure activity is that it has to be something that you *enjoy*. By all means, **try a bunch of different activities to find something that you really like**. Sometimes you may have to try something a few times to decide whether it is an activity you enjoy enough to do regularly.

You also have to consider the following:

- What are the physical requirements of the activity? (e.g. reading vs. skydiving)
- Can you do the activity during a flare-up? If not, have some alternative activities for times when you are not feeling so well.
- Is it an indoor or outdoor activity? If it's an outdoor activity and you are sun-sensitive, always remember to wear the appropriate clothes, use sun block, and try to avoid the midday sun.

- How much does the activity cost (e.g. walking vs. water-skiing)?
- How much time does the activity take?
- Does the activity require a lot of planning?
- Can you do the activity either with friends or alone?
- Has the activity been approved by your doctor? Make sure it has!

There are lots of options for your current (and future) state of health and lifestyle. Even if you are really sick, try to find enjoyment in activities such as reading or writing. You may consider learning a low-key hobby (like knitting) when you are well, because you will be more likely to continue this activity when you are experiencing a flare-up.

Once you've decided on a hobby that is appropriate for your lupus and your lifestyle, then do your best to stick with it. The key to doing this is to schedule your leisure activities along with everything else you have to do. Include "leisure-time appointments" in your calendar, just like you do for all your other appointments/meetings and commitments. When Jodie first met Jessica, she was already scheduling leisure time in her calendar, and protecting that time for herself. Initially, Jessica was surprised and amused by this, but she soon saw the value, and was inspired to do the same. **Taking care of yourself is important, so you might as well block the time in your agenda!** It might take some getting used to, but if you write it down somewhere, you will be more likely follow through with it. It's easy to let activities slide, especially when you are busy, tired, in pain, or just feeling down. Doing the activity will usually make you feel better, but be sure to listen to your body to make sure you aren't overdoing it.

I Need a Vacation...

Just the thought of a vacation can make some people instantly relax, and can make others instantly panic. Even though you are supposed to enjoy taking a vacation, it can still be quite stressful, and it can be even more stressful and complicated if you have an unpredictable illness like lupus. Still, **a vacation may be just the thing you need to relax, reenergize, and rejuvenate.** Taking a vacation can offer a real chance to truly enjoy yourself and what life has to offer. As we mentioned before, stress reduction is a key part of coping with your illness, and a vacation can be the ultimate way to relax, but in order to maximize your fun and minimize your stress, you need to choose the right type of vacation for you and your lupus. There are countless options to consider, ranging from "stay-cations" to cruising through the Mediterranean, but as a starting point, we suggest you consider the following aspects when planning your vacation.

Travelling: far and away

Pros: Travelling outside your country is very exciting. When you are far away, you can really get the sense that you have left your stresses behind, and it can be easier to disconnect from your everyday life, including your email and phone. It's very stimulating to be in a new place, and you can learn a lot of new things in a new country. There are also lots of options for your mode of travel, such as backpacking, camping, staying in hostels/hotels, preplanned bus/train tours, all-inclusive resorts, or taking a cruise.

Cons: These kinds of trips are usually more expensive and harder to plan, because you're unfamiliar with the country and the tourist options that are available. International trips can be longer, and you may not be able to take enough time from school/work. Travelling in another country (especially if there are language barriers) can be really hard and stressful. No matter the length of your travels, you will need to be really organized regarding your medications and health-care options. You have to consider that you may have a flare-up in a foreign country, which will not only be stressful, but could also be very expensive, and add to the length of your stay.

Cruisin'

Pros: Everything you need is right there on the boat, such as your meals and entertainment; plus, you stay on the boat, so you don't have to re-pack. You also have lots of options to relax, and there are different cruise options based on location and length of tour. You can hang out by the pool, read a book on the deck, or go on a few day trips. You can see many different places in a shorter amount of time. There are usually doctors/nurses on the ship to help you if you experience any health issues.

Cons: These trips can be quite expensive, and you may not enjoy the same cultural experience as you would while travelling far and away. Most day trips are organized in popular (i.e. busy) tourist locations, and are only for a very short time. If you are sun-sensitive, you may be limited with regard to the amount of time you can spend on deck while you are cruising.

All-inclusive resorts
Pros: Everything you need is right there, such as your meals and entertainment. As with cruises, you also have lots of options to relax, such as getting a massage, or hanging out by the pool, or the beach. You can also do day trips if you feel like getting away from the resort and/or want to see some local cities/sights.

Cons: These vacations can be expensive, although you can often get great deals if you are flexible regarding departure dates. You may not get the true cultural experience, as these types of resorts are often far away from the locals.

Backpacking
Pros: This type of trip is usually one of the cheapest, and you will definitely get a true cultural experience. You will meet lots of new people and see lots of cool things. It will be very exciting and filled with adventure! It will also make you feel very accomplished, even though you have an illness like lupus. You can also travel on your own schedule, or join a package tour, and pre-plan (or not) as much as you like.

Cons: This is not the kind of trip for the faint-hearted or anyone who isn't prepared to travel light. Because you will be carrying all your gear on your back for a long period of time, you will need to be physically strong, and your lupus should be under control. Backpacking can be somewhat unpredictable with regard to sleeping arrangements and the people you meet, which can be very stressful.

Camping

Pros: This type of trip is much cheaper, and can be easier to organize. If you undertake a camping trip, you will undoubtedly feel great, knowing that you did something so adventurous in spite of your illness. There are plenty of options for camping, ranging from grabbing a backpack with a few of your belongings and heading off into the woods, to booking a campground at a provincial/state/national park a few months ahead of time and driving to your site. No matter the option, being surrounded by nature can make you feel very connected and at peace, and give you new perspectives on your life and your lupus.

Cons: Camping can be expensive if you don't already have the necessary equipment. It can also be very unpredictable with regard to weather and encounters with wildlife. You may also need to be creative with your meal planning by preparing meals that are not only easy to make, but nutritional as well.

Short trips

Pros: Getting away for the weekend or just a few days can be very relaxing, and can really help you recharge your batteries. For example, you can go to a bed and breakfast for a few days, or an exciting city. These kinds of trips can be fairly cheap because they are shorter and closer to home. Short trips might also be less stressful, and may require less planning compared with a lengthy international trip. You just need to pack a few days' worth of meds and some clothes, and you're off!

Cons: Staying fairly close to home may not be as exciting or exotic as venturing far and away. In addition, when you are far away, you can really get the sense that you have left your stresses behind, which can help you to relax more deeply.

Trip tips

We both love to travel, and have managed to do some really cool trips while having lupus. Here are a few tips that we can offer based on our own experiences in all the different travel categories mentioned above.

- Inform your doctor, either by phone/email, prior to departure. Give details like the destination, and how long you will be away for.
- Get all your prescriptions filled. It's helpful to have a few pillboxes and to prepare all of your daily meds in advance. Take a few extra supplies as well, just in case you encounter any delays!
- If you are flying, pack your meds in your carry-on luggage so that you will have your meds with you if your luggage gets lost (trust us, it happens!). Also pack a letter from your physician outlining your diagnosis, your list of medications, and their purpose. This will enable you to deal with any questions from authorities searching your bags.
- Buy medical insurance if you are leaving the country. You might already have a plan through your job/school or credit card, but even so, check your current level of coverage before leaving. You can also buy additional insurance from your travel agent or airline if you need to upgrade.
- Write down some emergency numbers for all the places you will be visiting (like the nearest medical facility).
- Be sure to pack lots of sun protection (sunscreen/hats/long-sleeved shirts)
- Carry some over-the-counter medication that does not interact with your lupus-related prescriptions for other issues like the flu, colds, allergies, etc.
- Take lots of breaks during your vacation. Sure, it may seem tempting to see and do everything, but it's not worth it if you trigger a flare-up. Plus, a big part of taking a vacation is relaxing and enjoying the moment.
- If you are travelling with others, make sure that at least one person knows that

you have a medical condition.
• Relax!

Stay-cations?

A really cool thing to do for a vacation is to not leave your house at all. "Stay-cations" have become really popular, and are a great option if you have lupus. The benefits are obvious; they're cheap, convenient, and easy to plan. All you have to do really is book off from work/school and take it easy. Do not use your stay-cation time to knock things off your "to-do" list. Instead, try to disconnect from some of your usual routines, like email/Facebook™. After all, you might not do those things if you were away, right? The key to leisure time and vacations is taking some time to really relax, and it doesn't really matter where you go (or don't go).

Overall, the point of all the suggestions in this chapter is that your life doesn't have to be less cool, or less interesting, or less fun now that you have lupus. You can still have a fabulous and exciting life, and do all the things you want to do. We are proof of that! Jessica has traveled all over the world and spent time living in different countries, all while managing her illness, so never think there is something you can't do or somewhere you can't go. There are so many wonderful places to explore and so many ways to do it. So, get out there and live your life! Yes, you do need to be prepared, flexible, and creative, but you never have to give up your fun.

STRESS & ENERGY

Stress: The Good, the Bad, and the Ugly

We totally understand. We all have a lot of things that we need to do, like school, work, and housework. Those of us with lupus have to add on the responsibility of managing our illness. You can easily start stressing when you think of all the different things on your "to-do" list, but stressing is only going to make things worse! Not only do you waste time not getting anything done, but stressing could also make your lupus symptoms worse, not to mention the effect stress can have on our sleeping patterns. So, as much as stress is a part of our lives, it is especially important to manage it when you have lupus!

Stress is a word we hear a lot, and often in the negative sense, but stress can also be positive. We need a little stress to be productive in life. If we did not have any worries or goals in life, we would not have any reason to get anything done! It is only through experiencing a little stress that we accomplish a task. It is by doing things (especially challenging things) that we are able to create happy, memorable moments and develop confidence in our abilities.

Not only can stress be both good and bad, there are also many different types of stress. There is the stress of having a lot of things to do, but there is also reactive stress and emotional stress. Reactive stress happens when we constantly think about something that has happened in our lives, or something that is about to happen. We break the event down into minute detail, and are then overwhelmed by all the things that went wrong (or could go wrong). For example, when you break up with a boyfriend, or are preparing for an exam, you think about all the things your boyfriend said while you were breaking up, or you worry about how your mind will go blank in the middle of the exam, causing you to fail. All of this worrying leads to stress, which often becomes so overwhelming that it starts to control our lives. Taken to extremes, this can stop us from participating in activities, even those that we would normally enjoy. We offer some suggestions for stress management later in this chapter.

For those of us with lupus, reactive stress can happen while we are awaiting a diagnosis and are worried about what illness we might have that has been causing all our symptoms, or, once you have a diagnosis, worrying about how you will still manage to do the things you enjoy despite your lupus. If you are stressed about your future with lupus, know that this is normal. We have all struggled at some point (and sometimes still struggle) with these feelings associated with our illness. Learning to deal with the stress is something we have all had to face and, as a result, it has made us stronger and healthier.

Emotional stress occurs when something terrible happens in our lives, such as a death in the family or being diagnosed with lupus. The emotions we experience can lead to challenges with getting all our usual tasks done in our life. We can be so sad and angry that we cannot focus on other things, and then our "to-do" list can grow. Emotional stress can lead to reactive stress, the stress of having a lot to do, but it doesn't have to be that way! When Jodie was diagnosed, she did not experience extreme emotional stress. She knew that there was a reason why this was happening to her, and was able to appreciate that positive things would happen because of her being diagnosed with lupus. These positive things (like working in health care) have happened not only to her, but also to her family and friends.

No matter the type of stress, there are good ways and bad ways of coping. One good way is to reach out to others for help. This can be really hard to do, because many people don't want to admit that they are overwhelmed and need help, however, it is really important to ask for help when you need it. Don't be afraid. If you are wondering whether you need help dealing with something, you likely need some sort of support. Your friends and family love you, and don't want you to be stressed out. Yet, as we discussed in the Relationships chapter, help from others is only truly helpful *if it is the type of support you need.* So, when reaching out for help, be sure to let the other person know exactly what you need. Do you just need them to listen while you make a plan to tackle your "to-do" list? Or, do you need them to help you put a situation into perspective so that you can reduce your reactive stress? Sometimes it's hard to know what you need from other people, in which case the most important thing is to start talking, and then hopefully you will realize what you need.

There are also things you can do on your own to reduce your stress. One thing you can do is to permit yourself to feel whatever emotions you are experiencing, but then to move forward and let go of those old feelings. It is absolutely normal to experience a complete range of emotions in your life, but it is equally important not to let any single emotion totally take control of your life. Some people find it helpful to use a timer, and permit themselves to feel the negative emotions/stress for a certain length of time, and then move on with their lives (and all the wonderful things included in it) once the time is up.

Another key way to reduce your stress is to make a "to-do" list, and then rank the items on your list in terms of priority. Although seeing so many items on your "to-do" list can lead to stress, writing everything down and then prioritizing is a great way to manage your stress (and your time). If you truly have a very long list, or a very large task, try to break it into smaller chunks. For example, identify which tasks you are going to tackle each day of the coming week, and those that you need to get done within the next month. Perhaps you have to prepare for a big exam. In this case, break down the material you need to study into smaller, more manageable components. This can be easier to deal with than looking at one extremely long "to-do" list. Lists can also be very rewarding when you get to cross something off!

So, if you have class assignments and exams, you volunteer one night a week, work a part-time job, and have a birthday party to attend: (1) start with the concrete, and write down your class times and the nights you volunteer for the next month; (2) add in your shifts at your part-time job, and the date of the birthday party; (3) write the due dates for your class assignments and the dates of your exams; (4) back-track from the birthday party and, on the days that you are not working or volunteering, schedule time to prepare for the party; and, (5) divide completing your class assignments and studying for your exams over the remaining times. Remember to schedule some relaxation time for yourself, and some exercise time. Don't try to cram too much in: be realistic about what you can accomplish in one hour of free time between classes.

Jodie finds it extremely helpful to keep a calendar with deadlines for the next month/year, in addition to keeping a list of things she needs to do each day and each week. Your calendar on your computer/phone/tablet can be set up to send you reminders/alerts. There are plenty of other little things you can do that can be helpful. Have you ever thought of something you needed to do at home while you were at school/work? It may sound silly, but why not email/text or even call yourself at home and leave a message as a reminder? A similar tactic can be used if you find that you're unable to sleep at night because you're thinking about things you have to do, or are overrun with emotional stress. Keep some paper and a pen next to your bed and write things down. This helps your mind to address the concerns, realizing that they are important, and that they will be dealt with in the morning – not while you are trying to sleep.

The bottom line with stress: a little is okay, because it keeps us motivated, however a lot is not good, because it prevents us from getting things done, and can even make us sick! If you are constantly stressed out and start to experience negative emotions (like irritability or anxiety) and/or experience physical effects (such as insomnia or an upset stomach), you may benefit from speaking with a professional, such as your doctor, social worker, counselor, or the local distress line. You can manage stress – it does not need to control your life. There are lots of ways to deal with stress, so don't continue to suffer. You are not alone! Please speak with your rheumatologist if your lupus symptoms keep reoccurring during stressful times in your life so he or she can review your medication, and/or provide other suggestions on ways to reduce the impact of stress on your lupus symptoms.

The Zen Lupus Patient

Speaking of your rheumatologist, part of what makes life with lupus more stressful is trying to balance your regular life with doctor's appointments, follow-up visits, regular blood work, etc. When Jessica was first diagnosed with lupus, her biggest stress was actually managing her new life as a lupus patient! Again, the best way to deal with all of these medical commitments is to list them on your "to-do" list (weekly, monthly, yearly). You can also take charge of your medical appointments by requesting that they be scheduled to suit your timetable. Whether this means scheduling them all on the same day to avoid taking more than one day off school/work or scheduling them on different days to balance your energy levels is entirely up to you. Another tip is to use your calendar (either electronic or paper-based) not only for keeping your schedule and "to-do" list straight, but also for reminders. If you need to schedule a follow-up appointment, but cannot do it immediately because the doctor is not scheduling that far in advance, write yourself a reminder note to call in a couple of weeks. Whenever you have your blood work done, as soon as it's completed, grab your calendar and add a reminder about your next test on the appropriate date. Jessica also suggests keeping all of your medical documents together in a file folder or box, and saving all your electronic records in special folders on your computer. She also found it helpful to use the same pharmacy for all of her medications, for three reasons: (1) the pharmacist got to know her; (2) the pharmacist was able to more accurately track possible interactions when new medications were introduced; and (3) the pharmacist could make more informed recommendations for over-the-counter medication. As you progress through your lupus journey, you will no doubt develop your own organizational tools to ease your stress, but we hope that these ideas will help get you started!

Keeping all your medical stuff in order also means knowing how to speak up for yourself. This can be difficult if you don't know all the ins and outs of the medical system, which means you probably don't know the exact questions to ask, but if you don't ask, you will never know. No question is a bad question. You are a part of your health-care team, so do not hesitate to let your doctor know your opinion and to share your feelings. For example, if you are not completely comfortable with your doctor's recommendations, let him or her know what you are thinking. Most doctors are open to discussing how to move forward with your treatment, and are willing to listen to your concerns (for example, you might be heading into a busy period at school/work) and take these into consideration when deciding on your prescriptions and dosages. After all, you are the patient! Think about it: you are more likely to follow doctor's orders if you were a part of the decision-making team! Conversely, you are less likely to follow your doctor's recommendations if you do not agree with them. So, take charge of your health by not only being good to yourself and balancing your stress, but by also being an active participant in your health care.

Sometimes, following your doctor's orders can be stressful, because they can be so complicated! So, here are a few suggestions to help keep you on the right track:

1. Speak to your doctor about your prescriptions, your preferred modality (pills vs. needles), and your preferred time of day for taking your medication. There may be a way to reorganize your prescriptions to make it easier for you to remember to take them, and to avoid the awkward situation of having to take medications in the middle of class or work!

2. Ask your doctor about different ways you can manage your symptoms. Many doctors are happy to refer patients for massage therapy to ease aching joints, and are becoming more open to alternative methods of management – as long as these do not interfere with your prescription medications. Just as we encouraged you to research what you can access with regards to health-care claims for your taxes (see the Money & Finance chapter), we also want you to be open to exploring all your options for health management.

3. Use whatever method works as a reminder to take your medication, and to follow other orders from your rheumatologist. We suggest having a weekly pillbox – some pharmacies even prepare medications in this format so you don't have to figure out what pills to put into which slot. Some people set alarms on their cell phones to remind them. Jodie leaves her pillbox out so it

is visible when she is eating her meals. Basically, do whatever works so you can stay healthy!

Energy Management

You might be thinking, that's all well and good, but what about the fact that you don't have the energy to consider trying the suggestions in this chapter? Think about it: your energy will likely improve if you try some of these suggestions, because the more you take control, and add both balance and structure to your life, the better you will be and feel. This is particularly important to those of us with lupus, because our energy levels can fluctuate so much. When you do not have a lot of energy, it is even more important to manage the little that you have!

In the meantime, how do you raise your energy levels? You need to consider a few things when trying to figure out how to do this: (1) What time of day do you have the most energy? (2) What time of day do you have the least amount of energy? (3) Do you go to sleep and wake up at the same time every day? (4) Do you eat properly? (5) Do you exercise regularly? (6) Are you taking any medications that are making you more tired? (7) How do you spend your time when you are not doing something you have to do?

If you are not sure about the answers to these questions, then take a week or two to track yourself in these areas. From there, you can make some positive changes in your life. A permanent change in your habits can take anywhere from a few weeks to a few months to seem natural, so stick with it! Of course, take your lupus activity into consideration. If you are super-tired, then maybe a session at the gym is not your best option, but a little exercise is good for everyone. As you read in the Staying Active chapter, exercise leads to more energy and better sleep, which in turn gives you more energy. It's a win-win situation.

Another thing you can do to manage your energy is to schedule in some time to rest. I know it seems kind of strange to actually include a "rest" appointment in your calendar, but it is so important to set aside some time to relax and rejuvenate. It is very easy to get so caught up in our hectic lives that we forget that rest is an important part of our day. Rest does not mean sleep (although sleep is crucial in helping you to cope with lupus), but actually taking time out and relaxing. During this relaxation time, you can meditate and/or reflect. Maybe you can combine your relaxation time with another light activity such as taking a bath or reading a book. Just be sure that your body is at ease and that your mind is at rest, and not processing a million thoughts at once. Even some quiet reflection or deep breathing for just five minutes will help calm your mind, revitalize your spirit and, yes, give you more energy.

We have touched briefly on the importance of getting sufficient sleep in other chapters, but in this chapter concerning energy, it is worth revisiting a few important points. Everyone needs a different amount of sleep. Most people need 6–8 hours per night to be rested and productive the next day. Yet, for those of us with lupus (particularly when it is active) we might need a little more than our usual 6–8 hours per night. We may also need a nap during the day to be able to keep going. This might be difficult for you depending on your lifestyle. Many of us like to go out at night, or have to stay up late to study. It's irritating to have to focus on getting lots of sleep when your friends can stay out all night and party, but sleep is a huge factor in controlling your lupus. You can still have nights when you have fun or get things done, but for the most part, you will really have to make sleep a priority in your life. Managing your stress, eating properly, and getting enough physical activity are all important contributors to a good night's sleep, but so is a good bedtime routine. Try to establish a calming routine that actually makes you want to go to bed. This helps you to develop positive associations with sleeping, which is very import-ant, because sometimes when you are having problems sleeping, you can start to become anxious about going to bed (which of course leads to more sleep problems). There is plenty of information available outlining the importance of maintaining the same routine in the evening to prepare your body for sleep. Likewise, there is information concerning the importance of not exercising or not eating too close to your bedtime, as well as not watching television or using your computer/tablet before you go to sleep. Some people even find that the temperature in their room makes a huge difference to the quality and quantity of their sleep. Most importantly, find what works for you, and then do the same thing every night, at the same time, to prepare your body and mind for sleeping time. If you find that you are not getting the amount of sleep that you need, and if you feel constantly tired as a result, please see your doctor right away. Be proactive about your health, and everything else will improve!

If your lupus is really active, you might need to reevaluate your priorities – if so, be honest and patient with yourself. It is most important that you get healthy again before tackling other items on your "to-do" list. For suggestions on managing your school/work, exercise, and relationships during a flare-up, please refer to the relevant chapters for tips that we have learned from our own experiences. We are both wishing you more energy to enjoy all of your activities in good health!

SPIRITUALITY

Meaningful Living

Spirituality means something different to everyone. Not all of us will think of ourselves as spiritual beings, however, we hope that this chapter will help to enlighten you regarding the different aspects of spirituality and its importance in your life with lupus. Keep in mind that this is not *all* about religion! **Spirituality is simply about seeking out the positive sources of support in your life, making peace with those negative sources you cannot get rid of, and doing away with those negative aspects that you can easily leave behind.**

It can be overwhelming to struggle with different aches and pains, the challenge of finding the right diagnosis, and then trying to understand the impact of your condition (and its treatment) on your life. Some of us will simply shrug our shoulders, acknowledge that we all encounter challenges throughout our lives, and make the best of it. Meanwhile others will be very anxious and stressed trying to understand the meaning of their diagnosis and why they have been specifically chosen to live with this chronic health condition, and will struggle to incorporate lupus into their life. These people will ask a lot of "why me?" type questions. No matter which group you are in, how do you make the best of your situation?

Spirituality is about having a good mind–body balance and a positive outlook on life. All the stress and struggles we face in our lives affect our health; our mind affects our body, and vice versa. You can feel more pain in your body when you are sad, just as you can feel more stressed when you have an upset stomach. There is more and more research outlining the mind–body connection, and the importance of thinking positively to have good physical health. Being anxious and depressed can actually make your physical symptoms worse! So, how do you change your outlook on life if you are struggling to see the world through rose-colored glasses? We suggest starting with the small things – like acknowledging the things that you can still do, the things that you enjoy, the things you are looking forward to accomplishing, the people who are in your life and who are supportive, and anything else that reminds you of the good things in life. **Optimism isn't necessarily about ignoring the negatives we all face in our lives, but about embracing the positive and working hard to turn the negatives into positives.** For example, Jodie firmly believes that she was diagnosed with lupus to make her a better social worker. Her personal motto is that there is a reason for everything. She has an improved appreciation for life, takes good care of her physical and mental health, and enjoys the simple pleasures in life – like reading on a couch that is drowning in sunlight! We understand that this can be hard to do sometimes, but it's really important to focus on the good things in life. A refreshing walk through the woods can help, or sometimes chatting with an uplifting friend can do the trick! Jessica has compiled a book of uplifting quotes, and she reads these positive messages whenever she is feeling frustrated with her lupus or other things in her life. Try to find what works for you. There are lots of books (both non-religious and religious) that can help if you need a little inspiration. If you are having a really hard time working through some of your negative feelings, we encourage you to speak with a professional, whether this is a counselor, your doctor, or your religious leader.

You may not always know the reason for your diagnosis, your struggle, or the impact your health condition has on your family and other loved ones. It is particularly difficult to find a reason when you are in terrible pain and unable to get out of bed. But, the plan, and the reason, will be revealed in its own time. Try to turn your diagnosis into a positive: maybe you learned to communicate better with your parents, maybe you gained self-confidence by managing your lupus well, maybe you want to help others through difficult times, or maybe, like us, you want to share tips you've learned by struggling through the hard times with other young people with lupus. These are all positive outcomes from living with a chronic health condition.

That said, do not let others influence your perspective on life. **We all have a different definition of quality of life**, and you will find your own with a bit of searching and thinking. Some people would say that Jodie's life is incredibly challenging, balancing her health with all of her other demands, but she is quite happy with her quality of life. Similarly, most people believe that people who need to use a wheelchair have a poor quality of life, but this may not necessarily be the case. So, be your own advocate regarding what is important to you to improve your quality of life, and make your diagnosis meaningful!

Religion

Most religions actually believe that everything in life happens for a reason, and this can be a very empowering motto to improve your outlook and appreciation of living your life with a chronic health condition. Jodie had drifted away from her practice in her early years of attending Roman Catholic mass on a weekly basis, and was struggling to understand how she could reincorporate religion into her life. Then, one day she met an ultra-orthodox Jewish woman who made a comment about admiring Lenny Kravitz, which resulted in a roomful of wide-eyed, open-mouthed stares towards this hyper-religious person. The woman continued, "What? I am religious, not dead!" This was the jolt that Jodie needed to encourage her to re-explore her Roman Catholic roots, something she continues to this day, and in which she finds great comfort. Evaluating the importance of religion in your life is pretty common for young people. You might end up asking yourself even more in-depth questions, because you are also dealing with the challenges of a chronic and life-changing illness. This kind of exploration is worth doing, because you may rediscover how religion can help you (as was Jodie's experience) or you may decide that religion is not giving you the support you need. Either way, you are learning which strategies can help you cope with your lupus, and what is important to your quality of life.

Religion can be a source of strength by providing reassurance that there is a reason for everything, that there is hope, that "someone" is watching over you and has an ultimate plan for your life. The power of prayer, both individual and in a group, can be very beneficial. However, religion can also be a source of punishment, if it leads you to blame yourself for not taking care of the wonderful body you were given, or to wonder "Why me?" in response to all your suffering. Further, some religions do not believe in certain medical conditions/ treatments. Organized religion may not be your thing, which is fine - you don't necessarily need religion in your life to be a spiritual person.

Most religions teach you to honor your body, which is something that generally happens quite quickly when you are diagnosed with a chronic health condition. You come to realize how important your body is to you, how every-thing is interconnected, and how little things can make a huge difference in your everyday functioning and happiness. Your medical team will also be very happy if you learn to honor and respect your body, to treat your body well with nutrition, sleep, exercise, and fresh air. Sometimes, we like to experiment (for example, by staying up later than usual and seeing how we feel the next day), and experimentation is a part of learning our limitations while living with a chronic health condition. However, ultimately we know what feels good, and for some, what feels good is being a part of a religious community. Whatever you decide, just make sure that your beliefs are helping you to heal, and making you feel better about who you are.

Living in the Moment

Spirituality is being comfortable in your own skin, being thankful for what you have, and living in the beauty of the moment. **We grow through every challenge that we face in life**, and living with a chronic health condition is one of those challenges. We may come to appreciate good physical and mental health more than others who have not dealt with the same ups and downs. We might appreciate a fine, warm day, a friendly visit with family we haven't seen in a while, a good telephone chat with a close friend, earning our degree, even if it took us longer than other people, etc. If you are struggling to come to terms with your diagnosis and are not yet comfortable speaking with someone about where you are at mentally, meditation can help. For those who are religious, meditation can take the form of praying, but it can also be a separate activity. Meditation can come through living in the moment and appreciating the small things, it can be doing a mundane activity while reflecting upon life, it can be doing yoga and letting your body speak to you, or it can be writing in your journal to try and straighten out your thoughts. Repeating positive words/sayings or mantras help Jessica to relax and gain new perspectives in tough situations. Even deep breathing counts! Meditation is whatever works for you to calm your mind, body, and spirit. There is no time limit on meditation. Some people can get lost in their thoughts for hours, while others benefit from a five-minute break in the middle of the day to help them keep going. We have so much to be thankful for, so don't let the hard days get you down! Keep forging ahead, and together we can make it through and thrive!

CONCLUSION

New Normal

It's amazing how quickly your life can change after having been diagnosed with lupus. We know, because we have been there. One minute, you're just doing your thing, living your life, trying to achieve your dreams, then the next minute you have lupus. Whether you wanted to or not, you've had to make a number of adjustments. Let's face it, you probably weren't ready to deal with many of the challenges, and there are more challenges to come. Most of these challenges were, and will be, unwanted. But you've done it! Not only have you survived, but you have thrived! You have done what you had to do. This is your new normal. You are now living well with lupus.

Your life is different now, but that is okay. There are things you can do now that you couldn't do before, you have a better focus on what is important to you, and you have a greater appreciation of your health. You may have reevaluated some of your goals, and created a whole new future for yourself. Lupus gives you the freedom to sort out your priorities and to discover what your life's purpose is.

Lupus now gives you (and only you) the freedom to choose a brand-new path. Your diagnosis offers you the chance to decide what you are going to do with your life, and to shamelessly pursue your health and happiness, even if on a slightly different path than the one you initially thought you would follow. Your unique situation offers you an escape from unworkable expectations that no longer fit into your life, and you are now free to let go of the guilt that may have accompanied those old patterns and beliefs. You can now pursue new paths (toward goals that you never dreamed of before!) that are both lupus-friendly and fulfilling. This is your new normal. Live your life to the fullest! Be fabulous (with lupus)!

APPENDIX

Good Resources
Lupus Foundation of America (LFA)
www.lupus.org

Lupus Ontario
www.lupusontario.org

Lupus Canada
www.lupuscanada.org

Alliance for Lupus Research
www.lupusresearch.org

Lupus Europe
www.lupus-europe.org

Lupus United Kingdom (has resources for youth!)
www.lupusuk.org.uk

Cool blogs
Despite Lupus
www.despitelupus.com

The Life of a 20-Something with Lupus
www.flowonlupus.com

Cindy Coney: Live Beyond Limits
www.cindyconey.com

INDEX

CPSIA information can be obtained at www.ICGtesting.com
Printed in the USA
LVOW04s2216060415

433475LV00033B/2223/P